THE DIET OF DIETS

The Diet that never disappoints!™

THE

DIET OF

DIETS

The Diet that never disappoints!™

DAVID REUBEN, M.D.

Other Books By David Reuben, M.D.

Everything You Always Wanted To Know About Sex But Were Afraid To Ask™

Any Woman Can! *Love and sexual fulfillment for the single, widowed, divorced, and married*™

How To Get More Out of Sex *Than you ever thought you could*™

The Save-Your-Life Diet *Proven protection from six of the most serious diseases of civilization*™

The Save-Your-Life Diet High Fiber Cookbook™

Everything You Always Wanted To Know About Nutrition™

Dr. David Reuben's Mental First Aid Manual *Instant Relief! ... from 23 of life's worst problems*™

The Quick Weight-Gain Program *Safe, easy weight-gain for every age and situation*™

Everything You Always Wanted To Know About Sex But Were Afraid To Ask™ ALL NEW EDITION

Psychiatric Hospital™

The Diet of Diets *The Diet that never disappoints!*™

The Chinese Secret *How to save yourself from breast and prostate cancer ... and enjoy sex like never before!*™

Table of Contents

Important Message

This book does not constitute medical treatment or medical advice. Do not undertake any medical program unless until you have had a thorough examination and consultation with your physician. As with any diet program, if at any time during the program you experience any discomfort or serious symptoms consult your physician immediately.

1

What They Never Wanted You To Know

About Dieting!

Please don't think of this as a "diet book"—because that's *not* what it is. A "diet book" is usually a gigantic list of things you can't eat and a microscopic list of the things you can eat. Whenever I've read through that kind of diet I've always wished I could switch those lists around and eat everything on the "no-no" list and forget the low-calorie rhubarb pudding. I always promised when I designed a diet program I'd reverse those lists and let everybody eat the yummy things and prohibit all the nasty things—including the low-calorie rhubarb pudding. Well, now I've done it and as you read along you'll see how I've done it and I think you'll like it. I've arranged things to keep your stomach happy and your mind serene.

That's another important point. Most diet books explain losing weight is as simple as managing your bank account. They point out losing weight is a matter of withdrawing more calories (by exercising) from your "calorie bank account" than you deposit by eating. It's a sort of "spend-more-than-you-earn" way of doing things. What they are actually promoting is an approach to your health that would land you in bankruptcy court—or prison—if you applied it to your finances. It doesn't make much sense, does it? It also gives us a clue as to why almost all standard diet plans ultimately fail. And knowing that makes it almost certain that this one will succeed.

There's something else to keep in mind right from the first page. This is not a "diet book" in the usual sense. You and I are going to do it differently. We're going to take a journey together. Like every journey we're going to start off slowly and get to know the terrain and learn how to overcome whatever small obstacles we find in our path.

We're going to have some adventures and some excitement and we're going to discover some fascinating new things along the way. When we finally come to the end of our time together, we're going to have had some unforgettable experiences that will stay with us forever and that will help us to feel better and really *be* better as human beings. And as a special surprise we are going to find a new and very special way of eating that will make the whole problem of dieting and overweight a thing of the past—permanently. It's called the "Eighth Module" and although you're not quite ready for it yet, believe me, it's worth waiting for.

Now please settle yourself in a comfortable chair and brace yourself for what comes next. Hold tight. Here it is. It is a new weight loss concept that virtually every diet book ignores and ironically, it is the most important concept of all. It is an undeniable fact of reality:

*Overweight is **not** a nutritional problem.*

In all the thousands of books published up 'til now—the diet lists and calorie-counters and careful menu preparation to eliminate fattening foods are just playing games. And "game" is the word for it. Any school-girl—and most school-boys these days—can tell you that a gob of ice cream will put more weight on you than a nice red apple. So a diet book that tells you to eat apples instead of ice cream is really underestimating your intelligence—to put it politely. You already knew that. You also knew that you'll get fat if you eat candy and cookies. You knew that bread and cake and spaghetti will make you puff up around the middle. But now I'm going to tell you something that will surprise you—but don't worry! All the surprises you'll get in this book will be pleasant ones—that's a promise!

You can eat all those things and not gain weight.

As a matter of fact you can lose weight comfortably and easily as you eat many of those things that were supposed to be forbidden. How can you do it? That's exactly what we're going to look at right now. There are some very important principles of nutrition that we are going to put under the microscope before we go any further. They're simple and well-known, so it'll just take a moment or two. Please read them carefully and remember them:

1. Your body weight is a direct result of the number of calories you eat minus the number of calories you consume
2. To calculate the effect a meal is going to have on your weight, simply add up the caloric value of each separate food item.
3. Starches and sugars, item for item, are more fattening than proteins.
4. Exercise is a vital part of any weight-reduction program.
5. When you are losing weight you have to be very careful to get enough vitamins in your daily diet.

Got them all clear? Good! Now you can forget them—once and for all! *Because they are all wrong! One hundred per cent wrong!* These are the five pillars of nutritional misinformation that have kept hundreds of millions of struggling dieters from achieving their goal of rapid and pleasant return to normal weight.

It's worth emphasizing the concept of "normal weight" because no one in this world was born fat. Almost all of us weighed in at between about five and eight pounds—give or take a few ounces. Those of us who gradually crept up the scales didn't do it by accident. There were hundreds and hundreds of pounds of chocolate bars and potato chips that went down the hatch before we got where we don't want to be.

Now let's plunge ahead and take on those "five pillars of nutritional misinformation" one by one. Oh, but first, I forgot to tell you something. Do you know how most "diet books" are written? It's supposed to be a secret but you should really know. The prospective author—who may often be a saxophone player or real estate broker by profession or simply someone who was really fat and who has temporarily managed to lose weight—goes out and buys five of the most popular "diet books" and reads them, sometimes not very carefully. Then he or she whips up a "new" book based on what they have "learned" from their instant course in nutrition. How do I know that? I know it for two reasons.

First, after a few double whiskeys, authors, like everyone else, are prone to confess their sins. Secondly, all you have to do is read the "diet books" and you see that they continually repeat the same mistakes, over and over again.

Now let's move on to those mistakes as we take on the "five pillars of nutritional misinformation". Incidentally, so that we can move ahead a little faster, let's take the first two at once:

1. Your body weight is a direct result of the number of calories you eat minus the number of calories you burn up.

2. To calculate the effect a meal has on your weight, simply add up the caloric value of each separate food item.

This bit of silliness has been accepted as the true revelation of traditional nutrition. It puts the marvels of human digestion and metabolism on the same level as the clankings and sputterings of a second-hand jalopy. Fill the tank, step on the gas, and away she goes? But that naive and mechanistic approach ignores the obvious. Your weight depends on what proportion of your food ends up stored as fat ("adipose tissue" does sound a little more flattering, I must say ...), and to a far lesser extent, deposited as muscle and connective tissue. And that in turn depends on three separate factors:

1. How much of the caloric value of a food item is available to your body. For example, if we consult one of those endless tables of caloric values we find the following information:

Onions: 1 cup 64 calories
Wheat bran: 1 ounce 64 calories
Margarine: 2 tsp 64 calories
Grapes: ½ cup 64 calories
Whiskey: 1 oz. 64 calories
Egg (boiled) 1 small: 64 calories

Now can you actually believe that your body is going to process and absorb these six vastly dissimilar foods via the same route? Hardly. To understand precisely what happens, let's take a fast trip through the digestive system and see—in a very general way—what happens to the food after it passes your lips.

As soon as you bite into something—let's say a slice of bread since everyone eats a bit of bread from time to time—an enzyme in the saliva in your mouth known as "ptyalin" begins the process of digestion, by breaking down the starches in the wheat flour. By the time the bread reaches your stomach it is in paste form and in your stomach other enzymes begin to process the protein and the rest of the components in the bread-saliva mixture. After anywhere from one to four hours of churning around and being digested in the stomach, the bread leaves for its next destination—the small intestine. But it doesn't leave the same way it came. Now the various food elements that made up the bread march out of the stomach in single-file. First the carbohydrates slide out, followed later by the proteins, and finally the sluggard of the party, the fats, make their way out through the lower gate of the stomach.

The next big phase of digestion begins in the small intestine as the liver shoots a powerful cocktail of enzymes known as "bile", via the gall bladder into the now-liquid mass of food that was once a slice of bread. Among other things, the bile emulsifies the fat in the bread— that is, breaks it into tiny droplets so that it is more accessible to the rest of the digestive enzymes. Then the pancreas squirts in a combination of powerful and extremely complex—and not well understood—chemicals to finish the process of digestion.

It's important to emphasize at this point that most of what I have been describing is in a combination of wishful thinking and fanciful fairy tales—taken directly from the most-respected text books of medical nutrition. No one really understands any of what has gone on up 'til now although very few—if any—scientists will admit that in public. If you want the proof, here it is: no "expert" in nutrition at any of the multi-million dollar nutritional research centers so far has been able to duplicate a single one of even the simplest of the digestive enzymes. If your doctor ever prescribes enzyme tablets to aid your digestion, he will be giving you an extract of ox bile taken from the guts of dead cows or perhaps a little something whipped up from ground hog stomachs. Would you be surprised if I told you that exactly the same remedy was prescribed for Alexander the Great? And that it probably didn't help him that much?

The point here of course is that "scientific" knowledge of digestion is at best rudimentary. But compared to that, our understanding of absorption is virtually non-existent. I'll give you a general idea of what we know and then you'll see how badly off we are. Basically both water and alcohol can be absorbed from the stomach. Fat, protein, and carbohydrate are then absorbed in the small intestine. From there they pass directly to the liver and—that's when the heavy iron door of ignorance slams shut. The reference books start to say things like:

"Protein apparently cannot be synthesized from other foodstuffs."

"Whether or not fat can be transformed to carbohydrate, however, is still debatable."

"By very complex and not completely understood processes, fatty acids and glycerol are converted into ketone bodies, and the ketone bodies are further broken down to liberate energy with the production of CO_2 and H_2O."

Pretty unimpressive, isn't it?

But let's not spend too much time on the great unknown of food digestion and absorption. Let's press on to calories. Everybody knows about calories—at least everybody talks about calories. What is a calorie?

Well, a calorie is simply the amount of energy that a particular item of food contains and when you eat it, you stoke your body with that amount of energy. If you don't "burn" it up, it gets turned into fat and then you find yourself hanging around bookstores buying diet books to try and find out what went wrong.

The first thing that went wrong is that the whole calorie business is a perfect example of just what we've been looking at. Actually what most people calculate as a calorie is about one thousand times too small. The standard unit of measurement is a "kilocalorie" which is a thousand times bigger than the little ones. When someone says, "I only eat 1500 calories a day", they are really confessing to 1,500,000 calories daily or about 500,000 per meal. It doesn't really matter than much but it gives you some idea of how far off the mark the standard concepts of nutrition are. Let's press onward.

Those handy little calorie charts that dieters and diet books are so attached to—did you ever wonder who made them up? Brace yourself. Shortly after the death of Beethoven or just under 200 years ago, some intrepid researchers began burning individual items of food in big metal boxes, submerged in pools of water. They then measured the amount of heat given off and assigned that caloric value to the food. Those numbers, along with the music of Beethoven, have become enshrined in history. You would do better planning your menus on the basis of the Fifth Symphony than on the wild numbers of a Medieval calorie chart. Oh yes, there's one other little problem: these caloric values only apply if you habitually digest your dinner by sealing it in a metal box, sinking it in a tank of water, and then setting it all on fire with a big electric spark.

But it gets worse. The whole theory of weight reduction being used in clinics, hospitals, and doctors' offices around the world is only based on those figures. Here is the official tally:

1 gram of protein burned in a metal box produces 5300 calories
1 gram of carbohydrate burned in a metal box produces 4300 calories
1 gram of fat burned in a metal box produces 9500 calories

Very scientific and very impressive. Now let's have a peek at the real world. If we re-calculate the energy value of food by measuring what actually goes in within the living body of a human being we come up with these totally different figures:

1 gram of protein burned (metabolized) in your body produces 4100 calories
1 gram of carbohydrate burned (metabolized) in your body produces 4100 calories
1 gram of fat burned (metabolized) in your body produces 9300 calories

Huh? Let's ask the researchers what went wrong with their measurements. Here's the answer, taken from a classical reference book:

"The slight difference is probably due to failure of absorption plus a small experimental error."

What? Errors of two per cent for fat, five per cent for carbohydrate, and then a whopping *twenty-nine per cent* error for protein can be brushed off on "...failure of absorption plus a small experimental error"? Let us fervently pray that these same scientists never do any brain surgery:

"You know, we're really terribly sorry. It was rather awkward, I'll admit. It seems we removed a tiny bit too much of your mother's brain during the operation. Actually we only took about twenty-nine per cent more than we intended. Of course, she was getting on in years and the slight difference was due to a small experimental error ..."

There are other problems as well. The rate at which your food is utilized ("burned up") is strongly influenced by drugs, digestion, exercise, illness, mental state, climate, as well as the type of food that you eat. It is a fact—although obviously not a well-known fact—that radishes and cabbage can slow the thyroid gland and tend to make you put on weight although your food consumption may remain the same. And as a final blow to the "calories-in-calories-out" theory, there is a sensational metabolic explosion in our bodies several times a day! None of the traditional nutritionists have ever been able to explain it. Although it's tremendously important in every weight reduction program, you have never seen it mentioned in any weight reduction book ever published! Here it is now for the first time: It goes by the cryptic initials of "SDA" which stand for the cryptic terms, "Specific Dynamic Action". This is how it works:

The next time you are feeling a bit chilly when it's time to sit down to a meal, don't put on a sweater. Just pull your chair up to the table and eat. Within a few moments you will actually begin to feel warmer and if it is a heavy meal, you may actually have to open a window. It's the same thing that occurs when we have a snack on a cold afternoon.

The simple act of eating produces a sudden burst of heat or metabolic activity that can actually make us perspire. The rate at which our bodies are utilizing the food suddenly leaps up as much as thirty per cent over the normal metabolic rate! What's the scientific explanation? No one knows! It happens to the 7 billion plus people on this planet about three times a day every day of the year and none of the tens of thousands of nutritional experts has the slightest idea why. Gives you a lot of confidence in the calorie theory, doesn't it?

Now if we refer back to our list of six different food items each containing the same 64 calories (actually 64 thousand calories as we know by now ...) we can see them in a different perspective. It is almost impossible to believe that your body is going to make the same use of cooked onions, an ounce of ethyl alcohol, a boiled egg, 2 teaspoons of mixed fat, a handful of grapes, and an ounce of wheat bran. I can assure you that each of these will have a very different and very specific physical and psychological effect. Just as important they will have a totally different result as far as your weight is concerned.

There is another factor just as important and just as neglected. It's the effect one specific type of food has on the absorption of another type of foods that you eat at the same time. If you eat carbohydrate at the same time that you eat fat, is the absorption of the carbohydrate increased or decreased? If you sluice chocolate syrup all over your vanilla ice cream will the combination of sugar and fat put on more weight than if you eat them individually?

The ivory tower scientists who burn food in iron boxes say "no", but millions of overweight people think the answer is "yes". We'll find out the truth as we proceed, but in the meantime, think about it. How many times have you eaten a combination of foods and have been surprised—either pleasantly or otherwise—at the result? Haven't you noticed that sometimes you can eat vast amount of Chinese food, including really fattening stuff which would ordinarily add pounds the next morning? But the next day you wake up trim and slim? And then just one red-white-and-blue All-American cheeseburger can make you fat and depressed when you reluctantly shuffle onto the scale the next morning. Those are strange and mysterious things and we'll find out much more about them as we stroll down the path together.

In the meantime it's really important for both of us to remember the next line:

When it comes to nutrition, there is no such thing as democracy. All calories are **not** *created equal.*

That is one of the most important principles of *The Diet of Diets* and that's why it's going to be easy and exciting to lose weight—and to stay slim *forever.* Your body is not a giant metal box that burns everything that you put into it. It is a tremendously complex and sensitive mechanism that knows exactly what's going on in almost every cell of your body at any given moment—awake or asleep. Take just one tiny example:

It's four P.M. and it's been a hard day. You slump down in a chair and pour yourself a cup of coffee. You've decided not to eat anything except at mealtime but you need the pick-me-up of a good cup of something hot. No cream, no sugar, just a cup of black coffee. A few moments after the first sip, the caffeine from the coffee hits your brain. Since caffeine is a powerful stimulant—that's why you're drinking the coffee in the first place—you feel a jolt of energy. But it doesn't stop there. Nudged by the chemical, your brain sends a message to the pancreas to squirt some insulin into the bloodstream. The pancreas obliges instantaneously and immediately the level of sugar in your blood takes a dive. In a few seconds you feel an emptiness in the pit of your stomach and a tiny bit of light-headedness—characteristic signs of low blood sugar. What to do? Well, there's a box of cookies right there in front of you—the cookies that you said you weren't going to have today. But now you feel unwell and you need relief. So you pop just "a couple" of the cookies into your mouth and within four or five minutes you feel "better". "Better" because the refined sugar and carbohydrate in the cookies have found their way into your bloodstream, rapidly counteracted the insulin and raised your blood sugar. Tiny receptors in very special and very mysterious cells of your brain detect the chemical changes in the blood and send the message to the cells in the lining of your stomach and the areas of your nervous system that have produced the sensation of light-headedness.

Suddenly everything is fine now and you can go back to work. Well, not quite. Because the heavy dose of sugar and carbohydrate has overshot the carefully-maintained limits of blood sugar concentration in your blood. That triggers more insulin, lowers the blood sugar again, sets off the alarm in those special brain cells and sends you back to the cookie box. As you go back and forth on this metabolic see-saw, drinking coffee and eating the cookies you swore never to touch, you finally realize that things are getting out of control. So the conscious part of your brain overrules the metabolic signals, you push away your coffee cup, stand up, and take yourself away from the temptation.

This is a scene that is repeated all over the civilized world—and a good part of the uncivilized world—twice a day, 365 days a year. For many people, it is repeated at least three additional times a day: at each meal—with various foods and various types of metabolic reactions. And remember, we have seen just one type of metabolic interaction:

carbohydrate / caffeine / insulin / blood sugar

In the course of a typical day, there are at least a dozen similar metabolic and food interactions that work relentlessly against the willpower of anyone who wants to lose weight or even maintain their normal weight. This is the type of problem that no traditional "diet book" and no traditional concept of nutrition can help you with.

Now let's move on to the third pillar of "nutritional misinformation":

3. Starches and sugars, item for item, are more fattening than proteins.

Although that fairy tale has formed the basis for millions of dieter's menus, just a quick look shows that it just isn't so. The reality:

100 grams (about 3½ ounces) of sirloin steak, a typical source of protein in traditional "diet books", weighs in at 487 calories with 19 grams of protein and no carbohydrates.

100 grams of baked potato in its skin, a typical source of starch, adds a mere 93 calories to your daily routine while offering two-and-a-half grams of protein and 21 grams of carbohydrate.

That's the moment of truth. Item for item and weight for weight unrefined—that is natural carbohydrates—are not more fattening than proteins. But it goes even beyond that. The typical sirloin steak weighs about one pound or about 5 times the weight of a baked potato. It's easy to eat a sirloin steak and then go on to the rest of the meal— including dessert. But if you were to eat five baked potatoes—that's the same number of calories as one steak – you'd be through eating. Now you don't have to eat five baked potatoes—but that's an example of how most diet books sell you down the river.

Now on to the fourth "pillar of nutritional misinformation":

4. Exercise is a vital part of any weight-reduction program.

Of all the fallacies of nutrition and diet, this one seems to be the most innocent. After all, exercise is supposed to be healthy and so is keeping your weight under control so it seems sensible that one helps the other. But it doesn't work that way.

Let's take a couple of short inspection trips to see why. First, a visit to your neighborhood gym. If you notice that most of the people who are exercising there are overweight. Next stop, your local zoo. Now, there's something interesting. The animals who exercise constantly in their wild state, such as tigers and wolves, maintain normal body weight in confinement. And the only weight control is their diet. Check with their caretakers and you'll be surprised to find the "caloric value" of their food is just about the same as they are in the wild—where they spent all day racing around. What's going on? A lot of things ... and exercise is a lot more complicated than any traditional "diet book" ever told you. We'll see the real answer as we move along.

That takes us to the "fifth pillar of nutritional misinformation".

5. When you are losing weight you have to be very careful to get enough vitamins in your daily diet.

That's a great way to sell vitamin pills. We've all noticed our friends mightily gulping pills as they desperately try to control their appetites and replace their "lost" vitamins. But there are two big problems here. First, downing vast amounts of vitamins, especially those of the B complex family, tends to increase your appetite. The more vitamins you gulp, the more food you want to eat. That's bad news when you're desperate to shed the pounds.

The other problem is obvious if we stop to think about it. When you eat less, you digest and absorb less. That's what you need vitamins for—congestion and absorption of food. So when you eat less, you need less vitamins. The proof? Easy. People on weight reduction diets almost never have vitamin deficiencies. As a matter of fact, hardly anyone in modern countries ever has a clinical vitamin deficiency—but we'll see more about that later on.

With all the misinformation and confusing concepts in "traditional" diet books, it's a miracle that anyone who reads them ever loses weight, much less keeps it off.

But *The Diet of Diets* isn't a "traditional" diet book. Not by a long shot. In the pages that follow, we are going to take advantage of all our knowledge of human nutrition, of all of our instincts as human beings, of all the tricks and techniques we can muster, to solve once and for all that terrible problem of overweight. And don't ever, even for a moment, let anyone tell you that overweight isn't a terrible problem. Every major fatal disease of modern society is either directly caused by obesity or made much deadlier as a result of being fat.

Heart attacks, high blood pressure, strokes, diabetes, and many forms of cancer are all either precipitated or made worse by ten, twenty, or thirty pounds of extra weight. *The truth is that thin people bury the fat people.* You can calculate your life expectancy in terms of how much excess weight you carry around with you. For the first ten extra pounds of weight that you carry after the age of forty-five, you increase your chance of dying prematurely by about eight per cent.

And then, it *really* gets scary. For every additional pound of excess weight, the risk of premature death increases one per cent! So, the average forty-five year old who is 15 pounds overweight runs a thirteen per cent greater risk of death than his neighbor whose weight is normal. And remember, we're only calculating the risk of premature death. The chances of developing some chronic illness are astronomical if you are overweight.

Ask yourself this question: which of your overweight friends doesn't suffer from one of these? Diabetes, frequent colds, lack of energy, chronic headaches, high blood pressure, stomach upsets, and on and on. The weapon that has killed the most people is not the hydrogen bomb. *It is the brightly polished one ounce weapon known as the dinner fork.*

Now we come to two important points:

1. It is absolutely essential for you to keep a normal weight per-manently—for life.
2. None of the traditional "diet books" know how to help you do that.

The only way to reach that goal—and avoid chronic diseases and early death is to find the secret to control our weight that is safe, effective, enjoyable, and permanent. That secret exists. It is *The Diet of Diets* and it begins on the first line of the next chapter.

2

The Great Adventure

This is the chapter where we set off together on the great adventure of *The Diet of Diets*. Before we cast off let's go over our final checklist:

1. Have your full length snapshot taken.
2. Make sure your scale is working accurately.
3. Go to the fridge and give away or throw away all those wonderful-terrible things that helped us to get fat in the first place. I don't have to mention them—you know exactly what they are and where they are.
4. Tape a sheet of paper to the wall next to your scale.
5. At the top of that sheet, write in large block letters—in *red*—these words:

    Being fat means being ugly
    Being fat means being sick
    Being fat means dying young
6. On that sheet write down the date and your weight every morning as you weigh yourself.
7. Take a deep breath.

Here we go!

The Diet of Diets is a carefully integrated program designed to make your weight loss easy, pleasant, and permanent. If you follow it exactly it will function automatically. You won't have to think about what you are supposed to eat, you won't have to juggle calories, you won't have any discomfort whatsoever. If you try to do it all yourself, making up you own menus, selecting your own foods, designing your own modules, you may make some exciting new discoveries but you may just fail to lose weight. It's better to follow *The Diet of Diets*. Now here's what we've both been waiting for—the list of the seven modules:

1. High Protein/Moderate Fat Anorexigenic Diet
2. Carbohydrate-loading Anorexigenic Diet
3. Ten-Meals-A-Day-Always-Full Diet
4. High Protein/Low Fat Instant Weight Loss Diet
5. The Always Springtime/Always Munching Diet
6. The Super-Protein Unlimited Diet
7. Red-White-And-Green Eat-All-The-Time Diet

And of course, "The Eighth Module" when we finally get down to our desired weight.

The next step is to select the module from the list of seven that you are going to start off with for our first week. Before you do that, just take a moment or two and review a few of the most important basic principles of nutrition. That will help us make some of the important decisions and give us a clear idea of exactly how each module is working to help us. I should mention at this point that the concepts of nutrition that we are going to review are at best educated guesses. Any nutritionist who thinks that he knows everything is the one that is barely beginning to learn what the subject is all about. The mechanism of turning a lettuce leaf into a cell of the retina of your eye, or converting chocolate ice cream into a brain cell, is so unbelievably mysterious that we can only hope to glean enough understanding to help us lose weight safely and effectively. I can assure you that we are going to accomplish that at least. So let us set off into the uncharted wasteland of nutritional theory and practice:

All the thousands of different kinds of food that we eat can be included in three basic categories:

1. Protein
2. Carbohydrate
3. Fat

Everything from cauliflower to caviar, from pumpkins to pheasant, from cow's milk to champagne, falls into one of those three categories. Every item of food that exists on this planet is a combination of these three basic food categories. Our digestive system is so designed that it can process any one of a million possible edible substances and convert them into chemical combinations that enable us to keep on living from day to day. It is possible to exist—even to thrive—on such diverse fare as snails, fungus, seaweed, roots, and snake meat. The capacity of our organisms goes far beyond the standard supper: "meat and 2 vegetables". Now let's have a look at these groups one by one. We'll check out protein first:

Protein is what we are made of—mostly. All of our body—with the exception of our fat—is principally protein. A protein molecule, which is the smallest particle of protein that exists, is very much like a string of pearls. In this case, each pearl is a substance called an "amino acid". That "string of pearls" can contain as few as 55 or as many as 200,000 or more amino acids. These chains of amino acids make up all the various proteins of our body including blood, muscles, hair, heart, eyes, and all the rest. That brings us to a very interesting question:

If we eat, say, the muscles of an animal, as in a slab of porterhouse steak, how does that get converted into our muscles? Obviously there is a difference in the type of protein that makes up the muscle tissue of various species. We certainly don't have the same kinds of muscles as a cow. The same question might be asked for heart. If we eat calves' heart, how does that protein get changed into the protein that makes up our heart?

That's a good question since it is clearly impossible to simply take the heart out of a calf and transplant it into a human being and make it work. The proteins involved are totally different so some magic has to occur to allow us to utilize the animal protein that we eat. Oh, yes, there's something else. We don't only eat animal protein. How does the vegetable protein, like soy beans, get into our muscles and tissues? Obviously no one is going to suggest a soybean transplant.

The answer is a fascinating one. Our bodies have a way of disconnecting all those little pearl-like amino acids from the animal or vegetable proteins and re-stringing them into our own personal type proteins. Much of our digestive processes that have to do with proteins are aimed at accomplishing just that. So when we eat a pork chop, our body breaks it down into its component amino acids then it takes those individual amino acids and strings them together to form a brand new protein—our own personal protein. According to the requirements of our body at that specific moment, we may string together amino acids to form white blood cells, kidney tissue, or liver cells. Pretty simple, isn't it?

I sense that you don't agree that it's quite so simple. Well, as usual, you're right. It turns out that all of our thousands of different organs and tissues and cells are made up of combinations of a mere 22 amino acids, put together in an infinity of different ways. But hang on, it gets even more exciting. Of those 22 amino acids, we don't even have to eat most of those in their original form. Our body can synthesize—that is, make from scratch—at least 14 of them. (Children can only manufacture about 12 of the 22 amino acids. You notice I say, "about 12 …" because nobody really knows for sure. These are the generally accepted figures—which doesn't mean that they are correct. But for the purpose of understanding what's going on, it's going to be all right.)

So even if we don't get all the 22 in our diet, we're still in good shape nutritionally—almost. It seems that there are eight of those that we just can't manufacture on our own. These are called the "essential" amino acids and they are eight in number. We really need these to make the vital proteins for our own bodies and we have to get them from the food we eat. We don't have to have them every single day—thank goodness—but we do have to eat them fairly often. Just for the record—you know, in case someone asks you on a quiz show, or something like that—the eight essential amino acids are:

lysine, methionine, leucine, threonine, valine, tryptophan, isoleucine, and phenylalanine

So we have to get each one of those individual amino acids fairly frequently in our diet—not just to be healthy—but to survive. Then our bodies "restring the pearls" and turn cow protein or pig protein or soybean protein into human protein.

People traditionally have thought of meat as the best source of protein—but like much traditional thinking, it isn't necessarily true. The entire amino acid business is a bit strange. For a protein in your diet to be utilized with maximum efficiency not only does it have to contain all eight essential amino acids but they all have to be present in sufficient amounts. For example, if you eat a slice of bread you will get all the essential amino acids in sufficient quantity—except for lysine and isoleucine. That's not good news since the protein value of the bread will be reduced in exact proportion to the amount of the missing amino acids. That is, if the bread is missing half of its proportion of even one essential amino acid you will only get half the value of the protein in the bread. It doesn't seem fair, does it? If there are eight workers on the job and one of them is lazy and only does half a day's work, then should the other seven workers only get paid for half a day? Certainly not. But, in the world of proteins, there are no trade unions and the essential amino acid that doesn't carry his share of the load drags all the others down with him.

The essential amino acid that doesn't hold up his end is known as the "limiting amino acid" for obvious reasons. But he can't really do as much harm as one would imagine because we can put him together with another slacker, who also only works half-time, and get almost as much out of him as if we had one good hard worker. In the case of that slice of bread where lysine and isoleucine are the culprits, if we just pop a thin slice of cheddar cheese on top, suddenly we have all the essential amino acids present and working for us. The value of the bread and cheese together in terms of protein is at least twenty per cent more than if we ate the bread and cheese separately. Wow! That's a whole new world! We have just discovered a way to make our protein go at least twenty per cent—and up to fifty per cent—farther for us just by making intelligent combinations. So all of a sudden, the limiting amino acid is no longer so limiting and one bad apple in the batch can't ruin it for the rest of us.

Big time proteins like milk and cheese and meat and eggs all have all their essential amino acids in attendance constantly and working full time for us. Does that mean that we have to eat them every single day of our lives? To be honest, some nutritionists would have us believe that. "Eat at least one animal protein with each meal", they grumble, frowning at us as if something terrible will happen to us if we don't.

Well, it would be nice if we could. But animal protein is dreadfully expensive—perhaps because everyone is rushing to eat it after being chided constantly by the "experts" in nutrition. Have you priced eggs and meat and cheese lately? Sorry, I didn't mean to bring it up but you know what I mean. And think of it this way, if we really needed animal protein so badly, what does the 50% of the world's population do that never eats meat? And has very little other animal protein in the bargain …

Now it's time to ask how much protein we need to consume in a day. The answer to that—as with all questions where money is involved—depends on whom you ask. If you ask the traditional nutritionists they will give you this fascinating little rule of thumb:

"Divide your body weight" (in pounds) by two and that gives you the amount of protein (in grams) that you must consume each day to be healthy."

What? Let's try it. But I hope you're sitting down. Suppose you weigh 150 pounds. That means that, according to this rule, you should consume a whopping seventy-five grams of protein a day!

No problem. You could easily get that from about 3 quarts of milk or a dozen eggs or about a pound and a half of steak (weighed after cooking) or two pounds of beans.

But the big question is, after all that heavy eating how would you be able to walk around? Sound ridiculous? Well, it is. The classical nutrition books massively exaggerate your protein requirements and overlook the fact that an overload of protein can cause serious damage to your kidneys and other vital organs. Of course there is more profit in selling protein than any other major component of your food—except for vitamins and we'll see the amazing vitamin story very shortly.

Instead of setting arbitrary and excessive figures for protein consumption, why not take it from the other perspective? How much protein does the average 150 pound adult use up in a day? That's very easy to calculate and in fact has been measured over and over again. The answer is about 23 grams. Since an adult is not growing rapidly—at least not upward—it would be logical simply to replace the protein that he has used each day. So if we add a little reserve, we might say that about 32 grams of protein daily would do the trick. That's a far cry from drowning yourself in seventy-five grams of very expensive and largely useless protein food. Incidentally "useless" is the right word because the protein that you can't use that day—everything above the 32 grams or so—goes right out in your urine. All that extra trouble and all that extra expense—it's a shame to watch it go that way.

Okay, that's about what we need to know about protein before we get down to the details of selecting our first week's module. Let's take a look at fats—as we move ahead.

Now everyone knows what fat is—whether it's on our dinner plate or on our tummies. We usually think of fat as bad—in general that's true but like everything else, fat has its good points and when it comes to *The Diet of Diets* we're going to be surprised at how helpful even fat can be.

From a physiological point of view, all fats are made up of two basic substances: glycerin and fatty acids. We're all familiar with glycerin—really a member of the alcohol family, answering to the chemical name, "glycerol". It's a common ingredient of soap, face cream, and cough drops. The fatty acids number about two dozen and have such names as linoleic, linoleic, and arachidonic. They are strung together in various combinations to make up the various fats in the world around us. For example, olive oil is one combination of fatty acids while the fat in our bodies is another assortment of fatty acids linked together. Incidentally, olive oil is really fat although we call it an oil. Oil is nothing more than a fat that is liquid at room temperature. That's about all there is to know about fat.

What's that? You don't believe it? You think there's more? Okay, I was just kidding. There is one other little detail. It's that business about saturated fats and unsaturated fats and cholesterol and all that kind of stuff. For a hundred years or more, the classification of fats into "saturated" and "unsaturated" was an obscure technical detail of biochemistry, of interest only to research biochemists. Now all of a sudden it's on every label in every supermarket. What's it all about? It's all about … nothing. It's what you might call "under-whelming". This is the way it works:

Fatty acids are made up of carbon atoms, oxygen atoms, and hydrogen atoms, all hooked together in various ways. Generally the carbon atom is at the center and the hydrogen atoms are all around it. If a carbon atom is attached to all the hydrogen atoms it can accommodate, then it is called "saturated". If there is still room for more hydrogen atoms to be plugged in, then the fat is considered to be "unsaturated". Usually saturated fats are solid at room temperature, like tallow and lard and chicken fat while unsaturated fats are liquid at room temperature like cottonseed oil or olive oil. That's about it. Except for the fact that saturated fats supposedly gives you ... c h o l e s t e r o l ...

Here's the scoop on cholesterol:

I don't want to get too deep into sociology—we'll leave that for another book—but it seems that every society needs a monster just to keep everyone tense and nervous. A couple of hundred years ago it was the witches that were going to do you in.

In some areas of the world, the Evil Eye is working day and night to make you miserable. In many parts of the Caribbean, it's the zombies that come out at night and give you the works. And in our fast-moving Space Age, where we supposedly have overcome all superstition and childish fears, it's: *Cholesterol!*

Hundreds of millions of men and women are obsessed with a chemical they have never seen, couldn't recognize even if it were spread on their bread (something they do frequently without even realizing it), and *actually couldn't live without.*

Most people have been carefully and deliberately mis-educated— "brainwashed" is a less genteel term—about the biochemistry and physiology of fats. They have been told that if you eat animal fats, you will build up deposits of fatty "cholesterol" in your arteries. Then your arteries will get all clogged up like the drain in your kitchen sink and you will die! Pretty scary, don't you think?

I don't think so because I know it's just a fairy tale. Anyhow, these folks obediently boycott animal fats, cut down their egg consumption, exercise madly, and die just as soon—or sooner—as those of us who know the real story. And here is the real story:

Cholesterol is *not* a fat. It is really an alcohol—you can tell by the "-ol" ending on its name. It is a natural and *essential* component of your body. You wouldn't live a minute if you suddenly had all your cholesterol taken away. You would lose—immediately—your eyes, your nerves, your brain, your ovaries or testicles, your liver and a few of the other organs that are so useful in everyday life. As a matter of fact, cholesterol is so vital that your own liver manufactures it every day. That's right. *If you don't eat enough cholesterol, your body manufactures what you need by itself. (If you have any doubt about this, ask your doctor to explain how the human liver synthesizes cholesterol if the patient doesn't consume enough.)*

If you fall for the "cholesterol fairy tale" and drastically reduce your intake of cholesterol, your liver has to work overtime to make enough to keep you alive. In fact before cholesterol replaced witches and dragons as the "enemy of society", all the respected medical text books carefully listed your required daily dietary allowance of cholesterol! Okay, I know what you're thinking. How come some people die with their arteries—especially the tiny coronary arteries that supply the heart—clogged with cholesterol? The answer is one of the few honest answers that you will find in the field of traditional nutrition today.

Here it is:

No one knows.

What we do know is that it has very little to do with the consumption of animal fats or vegetable fats. Some of the most respected researchers in the world believe that the culprit is probably over-refined carbohydrates, mainly white flour and white sugar.

The most often-quoted laboratory experiment to prove how bad cholesterol is was done way back in 1911 by a Russian researcher who fed purified cholesterol to rabbits. Guess what? They developed deposits of cholesterol in their little rabbit arteries.

Well, first of all, no one in the world voluntarily consumes 'purified cholesterol'! But even more important, rabbits are vegetarians and they never eat cholesterol in any form, much less the super-purified form they were fed in the lab. Oh yes, there's one other little detail. *Rabbits aren't people*, something that a generation of cholesterol-haters seems to have overlooked.

Here's some other things that they have also overlooked:

1. According to the cholesterol fairy-tale theory eggs are supposed to increase the cholesterol in your blood. In actual fact, it works just the other way around. The more eggs you eat, the more your cholesterol level drops. Why? Because you are getting enough cholesterol in your diet and your liver doesn't have to struggle to make what you need. In fact, when some volunteers ate a dozen eggs a day, their cholesterol level fell sharply.

2. If avoiding cholesterol in your diet was going to cut the incidence of heart attacks, the theory has had ample time to work. In the United States, between 1909 and 1973, the population cut their consumption of cholesterol-containing fat by thirty-seven per cent. If a reduction in cholesterol consumption was effective in reducing heart disease, over half a century of mass experimentation should be long enough to show results. Well, it did show results. In that period of time, the death rate from heart disease has INCREASED a mere two hundred and thirty-five per cent! So by sharply reducing their intake of cholesterol, these unwilling guinea pigs have died by the millions.

3. If cholesterol is really so bad, then reducing the blood level of cholesterol should be effective in preventing heart attacks, right? Then how come, in one large survey, at least eighty per cent of people who had heart attacks, succumbed with absolutely normal cholesterol levels?

4. There's another embarrassing fact the cholesterol boys don't like you to mention. Hundreds of millions of people around the world consume a lot of animal fat in their diets—usually pig fat or lard, which is supposed to be terrible for making naughty cholesterol. Yet in these societies, comprising most of Latin America, for example, heart disease is relatively unknown.

It makes you think, doesn't it? Well, it makes the cholesterol theorists think too. Lately they have come up with a new and "improved" story. Supposedly there is now a "good" cholesterol and a "bad" cholesterol. (For the record, there is now something called "High Density Cholesterol" and another something called "Low Density Cholesterol". The "High Density Cholesterol" is the "good stuff" and the "Low Density Cholesterol" is the "bad stuff". Just so you get good and confused the cholesterol theorists also refer to these goblins as "High Density Lipoproteins" and "Low Density Lipo-proteins".)

Supposedly the "good" cholesterol protects you against heart attacks and the "bad" cholesterol gives you a heart attack. So you should eat "good" cholesterol so that it can fight the "bad" cholesterol. What do they think we are, a bunch of dummies?

And now some of the very latest and most sophisticated medical research seems to indicate that the "good" cholesterol really isn't that good.

Sounds like it's taken right from the little book of fairy tales nursie used to read to us! Surely you remember the "good" fairies and the "bad" fairies? So, let's not lose any sleep about the cholesterol ghosties and goblins and things that go "bump!" in the night …

One other point. You may have seen the newspaper accounts of the medical journal articles describing how a "low cholesterol diet" lowers the incidence of heart attacks. It sounds fine in the newspaper but if you read the actual medical journal articles themselves, it's a totally different story. The so-called "low cholesterol diet" turns out to be a low-fat, high fiber diet basically vegetarian with very little meat and animal products. But the explanation is the high fiber not the lack of cholesterol! *That's the secret*. The high fiber part of the diet is what saves lives—the "naughty cholesterol" is the smallest part of the problem.

In the meantime we will see, as we proceed, that fat is going to play a very useful role in our weight loss program. As a matter of fact, you might even call it a "creative" role—but more about that later on.

Okay, the only remaining member of the "Big Three" nutritional components that we have to review is carbohydrate. Let's see what that's all about:

Down through the years carbohydrates have gotten a bad name in dieting circles. Tagged with the unappealing name of "starches", most reducing diets color them bright red for "danger" and warn you to eliminate them from your diet—if you want to lose weight. Like most everything else in the "unscientific school of weight reduction", that is an oversimplification. It is true that some carbohydrates are really bad for you—and it's just as true that some carbohydrates are your best friends.

What's the difference? Refinement. The key word is "refinement". And in this case it has nothing to do with breeding, manners, or education. When a carbohydrate is refined or processed it turns from our friend into our enemy. Take wheat flour, for example. A grain of wheat has three components in its natural state: the bran, the germ, and the endosperm. Most of the wheat flour consumed in the U.S. has been "refined". That means the bran layers, which contain the fiber plus vital vitamins and minerals, are removed and sold to feed chickens. The wheat germ, which contains more protein than beefsteak, is also removed and fed to swine. The endosperm, which contains mostly starch, is ground and packed in bags and boxes to feed us. Lucky pigs and poor us.

Unrefined wheat flour—a natural carbohydrate—is a wonderful food. Refined wheat flour—a brutally-stripped carbohydrate, is hardly worth eating. Just for the record, here's the comparison:

Refined wheat flour, when compared to whole meal flour, has:

27% less protein
76% less iron
60% less calcium
97% less thiamine (vitamin B1)
74% less potassium
50 % less linoleic acid
94% less pyridoxine
66% less riboflavin
78% less magnesium
57% less pantothenic acid

and significantly *less* of the following important natural nutrients:

phosphorus, manganese, copper, sulfur, iodine, fluorine, chloride, silicon, boron, inositol, folic acid, choline and vitamin E

Could you be thinking what I think you're thinking? All that doesn't matter because refined flour is "enriched"? But don't be fooled. Enriched only means stripping the flour of most of its nutritional value and then dumping in a few artificial chemicals that cannot begin to compensate for what was taken out of the original natural product. Specifically in the U.S., more than 24 vital nutrients are removed from the wheat before it is made into white flour and two artificial vitamins (thiamine and nicotinic acid) and a little iron are added to replace them. Together they replace about one half of those three nutrients that have been removed. They don't replace any of the other twenty-one depleted nutrients.

In general, the same tragedy applies to white rice compared to brown or unpolished rice, refined white sugar compared to natural sweeteners, and other over-processed and de-nitrified elements.

Well, we've covered the most important aspects of proteins, fats, and carbohydrates. Before we finish this nutritional review, we should take a glance at vitamins and minerals so that we know what we're dealing with when we really start the day-to-day eating on our seven modules. Let's go to vitamins first.

The definition of a vitamin is hidden in the letters of its name: "vita" "amine". It's nothing more than a made-up word indicating an amine which is any chemical substance that contains nitrogen and hydrogen plus the Latin word, "vita" which means "life". The name was coined by Casimir Funk, a Polish chemist who discovered thiamine or vitamin B1. He originally called his discoveries, "vitamines", later shortened to "vitamins". It all fits in when you known the story.

In terms of your daily diet, vitamins are extremely common substances that we require in almost insignificant amounts. Vitamins are so common that it is impossible to eat without getting a massive dose of them. In the real world, the closest we can come to eating something that doesn't have any vitamins at all is white sugar, white flour, and white rice. Our daily vitamin requirements are so small that they are measured in thousands and even millionths of a gram.

There are some vitamins we don't even have to consume since our bodies manufacture all we need. Vitamin D is made in generous amounts when sunlight shines on guess what—the *cholesterol* in our skin! Incidentally did you know that vitamin D is "irradiated 7-dehydrocholesterol"? Imagine that! And think about it when you take those vitamin D caps and give them to your kids.

Vitamin K is constantly manufactured in our large intestine. In addition we have immense stores of some vitamins. If you could totally stop our intake of vitamin E today—and fortunately you can't—when would you run out of vitamin E? In about eight years.

If you begin to suspect that our need for vitamins has been grossly exaggerated, you are right. We could fill a thimble with all the vitamins we need in one month and still have plenty of room left over.

Vitamins are one of the world's greatest businesses because they are common substances easily obtainable at low cost. Once they are made into tablets, they suddenly become very expensive magical potions which are supposed to cure everything. Actually the only thing that vitamins cure is a shortage of vitamins. That has been given the scare name of "vitamin deficiency".

Sounds good—very high class. "It's not that my brother-in-law is dumb—he just suffers from an intelligence deficiency." "It's not that I'm short of money. I simply have a cash deficiency." You see what I mean? If one were to have a vitamin shortage, then the logical solution would be to eat more foods containing vitamins, not take pills that are merely synthetic or artificial vitamins. (Don't worry about pills that call themselves "natural" vitamins. The processing required to put them in pill form casts a shadow on the "natural" aspect.)

Yes, I know. We all read about the terrible symptoms of vitamin deficiencies but you don't personally know anyone who actually had a proven vitamin deficiency, do you? No, neither do I. And neither do most doctors in the U.S. Your daily diet, no matter how awful, is so chock full of vitamins that unless you have a serious disease that prevents the absorption of your food, it is virtually impossible for you to get a vitamin deficiency. If you find yourself in that unfortunate situation, then no vitamin pill in the world is going to help you.

But what about the people who feel better after they take vitamins? Well, some people feel better after drinking a double whiskey or taking an aspirin tablet. That doesn't mean they were suffering from a whiskey deficiency or an aspirin deficiency. Human beings are strange creatures, as you may have noticed, and if they think something is going to make them feel better, then often it does.

A lot of people think that vitamin pills are going to make them better. Those are the folks that swear by their bottle of pills. So long as they can afford the cost—without getting a money deficiency—then they probably can't do themselves much harm. But for you and I, as long as we eat what's on *The Diet of Diets*, we will never have to worry about a shortage of vitamins.

That same state of affairs holds true for minerals, but even more so. Minerals are just what they sound like—things such as iron, zinc, calcium, phosphorus, iodine, and all the rest. They are found in natural foods in great abundance. But of course, it would have to be that way. The vast majority of the people on this planet have never seen a bottle of vitamin pills nor a mineral supplement and they never will. Yet whatever health problems they have do not spring from missing out on their daily iron pill. As a matter of fact, the folks that live to be 110 and 115 years old such as the Caucasians of Russia, the Hondas, and the Ecuadorian hill people, have never taken a pill in over a hundred years. If you eat anything approaching an adequate diet—and in all of the modules that we are going to use, your diet will be more than adequate—you will never have a moment's concern about vitamins or minerals.

I think that covers most of the most important areas of nutrition. Now let's turn the page and pick our first Module.

3

The Only Thing We Have To Fear

We are now going to dispose of the single greatest enemy of success on any weight loss program. It's the most imposing adversary that we are going to encounter. It's the one that's going to make the difference between winning and losing in the next few months of our lives together. So, we might as well smite our enemy a mighty blow once and for all—right now!

The greatest enemy of success on a weight loss program is—FEAR! As a matter of fact, there are "FOUR FEARS" that can sabotage every sincere attempt to lose weight. Let's get them out in the open once and for all so we can get rid of them. Here they are:

1. Fear of being deprived
2. Fear of being hungry
3. Fear of failure
4. Fear of staying fat

Sometimes even thinking about starting on a diet brings on a little quickening of the pulse, a little tension in the stomach (where else?), a touch of uneasiness. But it doesn't have to be that way. Let's take those fears one by one and banish them forever—and then proceed swiftly to Module Number One: THE HIGH PROTEIN-MODERATE FAT ANOREXIGENIC DIET.

Here we go:

1. Fear of being deprived

For almost everyone, food and eating are major sources of gratification, of sensual satisfaction, literally, a way to have "fun". If we take away most of the eating, then we think we are taking most of the fun out of our lives. That's why the anticipation of starting on a diet—for so many of us—brings on so much anxiety. It's as if we were going to lose one of the biggest pleasures of our daily life. You know how it goes—a hard day at work, trouble with the boss, things a little tense at home— and then we can sit down and have a nice big dinner and maybe two helpings of dessert and at least we had something good that day. Fear of being deprived is a realistic fear and all reducing diets—except for *The Diet of Diets*—really do deprive us.

2. Fear of being hungry

Nobody likes to be hungry. It's a bad feeling. No, it's worse. It's a terrible feeling. Being hungry is like being in pain—you have to pay attention to it. It is one of our organism's danger signals—telling us that if we don't do something about it promptly we are going to die. Fortunately the definition of "promptly" in most cases is a month or two—the amount of time we can live without any food at all and stay fairly healthy. But emotionally we don't think of it in those terms. If we miss two meals in a row, we start to get a little frantic—as if we will never see food again. It's simply that fear that keeps so many people from ever starting a diet and causes so many who have started diets to suddenly start eating ravenously again.

3. Fear of failure

It's amazing how many people never even start a diet simply because they are afraid that they will fail. So often they say things like, "What's the use? I go through all that suffering just to lose half a pound and then I gain it back between breakfast and dinner!" Hundreds of thousands of people have been condemned to a life of obesity simply because they are convinced that even if they do lose a little weight, inevitably they will gain it back again.

4. Fear of staying fat

So many men and women who are more than twenty-five pounds overweight suffer from a combination of resignation and pessimism when it comes to ever being thin again. They have all tried diets and they have tried all the diets—except for this one. Some of them are beginning to convince themselves that it is their destiny to be fat. Others look for clothes that will disguise their extra weight. Still others become so depressed that they immerse themselves in food and start down the path toward "hyper-obesity". These are the folks who will one day be 100 or more pounds overweight—difficult, but not impossible cases. For everyone who suffers from the "FOUR FEARS" and for almost everyone else who is just starting out on *The Diet of Diets*, the best module to begin with is **Module One**:

Module One immediately and permanently banishes each and every one of the **Four Fears** and makes the first week on *The Diet of Diets* a pleasant adventure rather than a week of sacrifice and suffering. It swiftly and automatically accomplishes the following:

1. It eliminates all *Fear of Deprivation*. On **Module One** you can eat as often as you want and in virtually unlimited amounts. You never feel deprived even for an instant. If you have the urge to eat, you can eat—and still lose weight.

2. **Module One** eliminates all *Fear of Being Hungry*. Because of the beneficial biochemical and physiological reactions that the module produces, hunger vanishes within the first hour of starting the diet! As a matter of fact, that's the only criticism anyone has ever had of **Module One**. Occasionally someone will remark:

   "But I'm used to starving to death when I'm on a diet! It's such a funny feeling not to feel hungry at all. It seems almost immoral!"

   Well, if you love to suffer when you're on a diet, then maybe you'll want to stick to the old-fashioned ways of trying to lose weight. You don't think you want to do it that way? I don't blame you.

3. With **Module One** there can be no *Fear of Failure* since there is success from the first day. Everyone who has tried reducing

diets before immediately senses that **Module One** is something completely different from anything they have ever done before. The lack of hunger, the feeling of being in control, the sense of well-being that **Module One** produces immediately makes everyone who tries it optimistic and eager to continue.

4. **Module One** is the perfect answer to those who suffer from *Fear of Staying Fat.* As one patient expressed it:

"From the second day that I was on *The Diet of Diets* I knew in my heart that I would never have to worry about being overweight again. I couldn't believe that I'd finally found a way to take off weight at the same time I was eating as if I were trying to put weight on!"

Module One gives people a feeling of power and control over themselves that they have never experienced before.

If **Module One** is going to work for you exactly the way it should, you have to do your part. If you're really serious about losing weight—and I'm sure you are or you wouldn't have traveled this far with me—then you're going to want to do everything you can to help yourself and nothing to hold yourself back. Here are a few simple suggestions that will go a long way toward making this the most enjoyable diet experience you have ever had in your life:

1. Since **Module One** is a diet where you can eat all you want, don't try to prove how much you can eat. Don't try to beat the diet. If by tremendous effort and concentration you manage to force so much food into your stomach that you overcome the diet, you will be the loser. Put yourself in tune with **Module One**. Go with its rhythm and you will be amazed at what it does for you.

2. When you finish a recommended meal on **Module One** if you feel that you'd like to eat more, of course, you can eat more. But to help the diet work for you, *wait thirteen minutes by the clock.* The purpose of waiting is not to keep you hungry but to allow **Module One** to produce its beneficial effects on your body. The foods that make up **Module One** have to reach your stomach, be digested, pass to your liver, and send the

signals to your brain that eliminate both the physical and emotional feelings of hunger. If you rush to eat more, you can overwhelm these very delicate biochemical responses and make life harder for yourself by not getting the maximum benefit from **Module One**. Of course, **Module One** has some built-in safeguards to prevent this from happening, but it's much better if you work with the diet rather than against it.

3. Eat slowly and leisurely. If you do it that way, you will allow the first bite of your meal to initiate the essential biochemical reactions. That way, by the time you get to the last bite, you'll often have to struggle to finish it.

4. Remember, with **Module One** you can eat all you want. So you don't have to rush, you don't have to panic, you don't have to worry. For the very first time ever you have complete and absolute control over your eating and your weight. Enjoy it!

5. *Be sure to drink enough water.* Our bodies are 67 per cent water and every chemical reaction that occurs within us requires the presence of water. Your blood is 90 per cent water and your urine is 97 per cent water. You have working within you, twenty-four hours a day, 365 days a week, two gigantic water filters known as kidneys. Every day of your life, your blood is passed through these filters and the impurities and toxins that have built up in your blood are filtered out and later passed in the urine. The greatest single bit of harm you can do to your body is to not drink enough water. If you deprive your body from water the kidneys can't extract the poisons from your bloodstream and the concentration of those dangerous chemicals relentlessly increases in your body. How strange it is! People who empty their garbage cans as soon as the tiniest bit of garbage accumulates, allow their body to be choked with dangerous "body garbage" just for the lack of a few extra glasses of water a day.

With *The Diet of Diets*, it is even more important to drink abundant water since we are interested in breaking down fat tissue and eliminating it. The primary pathway to eliminate those dissolved fatty breakdown products is the urine—dissolved in water. Please be sure to drink at least *eight* glasses of water a day, no matter how much tea or coffee or sugarless lemonade you may consume otherwise. If that seems like a lot, here's the explanation:

We need at least four glasses of water a day just for the basic housekeeping of our body. We lose that in sweat, feces, urine, and general evaporation. If we drink another 4 glasses, that leaves us with a meager quart to handle everything else. That's the least we should consume and if we can sneak another glass or two in during our waking hours, we will be doing ourselves a favor . You can tell when you are on the right track when your urine is perfectly water-white, with no yellow pigmentation at all.

Of course, we aren't going to overdo our water consumption either. Twelve or fifteen glasses a day may be a bit too much although our bodies can safely handle about one quart per hour of liquid consumption. Obviously we're not going to drink anything like that! As usual, we're going to do everything within reason. Incidentally, as an added benefit, we will find that our liquid consumption helps our diet to keep us satisfied and contented.

With these general concepts to guide us, I think we're ready to launch **Module One**.

I know. What have we been waiting for? When are we going to get down to the actual menus and portion measurements? The answer to that is simple: *There aren't any!* I promised you a module where you could eat all you wanted and that means no menus and no portion measurements! (For your convenience, there are some simple and delicious recipes in the Chapter entitled, "Some Simple And Delicious Recipes".) But we will have to do a little bit of studying together so that we are well-briefed before we start off on such an easy and enjoyable diet. Here it is, **Module One**:

Eat as much as you want, anytime, of any of the following foods:

1. Any kind of FRESH meat.
2. Chicken, turkey, duck, goose, and any other kind of fowl.
3. Any type of fish.
4. Lobster, shrimp, crab, oysters, clams, and any other shellfish.
All right so far? Wait, it gets better:

a. Do NOT remove the fat from the meat or poultry. Eat the poultry with the skin—that's very important.

b. Please try to FRY everything that you eat on this module—within reason of course. (Don't fry the lettuce or the tomatoes—unless you happen to like them that way.) Use as much fat as you want but be generous.

What else can you eat besides meat, poultry, fish, and seafood? Well, that's a pretty good start. Let's see what else we can come up with:

5. Cheese—almost any kind of cream cheese, cottage cheese, cheddar, gouda, edam, or Swiss cheese. You should avoid any "processed cheese" because you don't know what's in it. "Processed cheese" is generally a combination of various kinds of cheese ground up with other assorted ingredients and then melted and poured into a mold to harden. You won't miss it.

6. Of course you can have cream—either sour cream or fresh cream.

7. Yogurt—but make sure it is plain, unflavored, unsugared, natural yogurt.

Spices and condiments? Sure. Any of the following:

1. Pepper

2. Mustard

3. Any natural spice such as oregano, thyme, rosemary, garlic, etc.

4. Fresh lemon juice anytime on anything.

How about beverages? No problem. As much as you want anytime of the following:

1. Tea—with cream, please. No milk or sugar.

2. Coffee, the same way. Real cream, no milk or sugar.

3. Carbonated water—unflavored and unsweetened.

4. Mineral water.

I can see the question forming on your lips: "What about diet soda pop made with artificial sweeteners?" You know, I don't really think they're a good idea on a diet. They are chemicals and I think we fool ourselves when we use them. There is no doubt that they are sweet and they sometimes increase our craving for sugar. On *The Diet of Diets* you won't miss them and we're all better off without them.

How about some vegetables? We won't have much variety but you can have *lettuce and tomatoes* as much as you want—so long as you use a generous amount of real old-fashioned salad dressing on top. That dressing should be mayonnaise or simply half olive oil and half vinegar shaken together.

Too good to be true? No. It's true. **Module One** is a very carefully designed, very carefully structured, and very carefully tested diet. It has been in use for over 1500 years and millions of people are on it permanently with no ill effects whatsoever. Now there are some things that we aren't going to eat on this diet but I assure you that you won't miss them at all. They include the following:

1. *Salt.* The food that we are going to eat has a fair amount of natural salt in it already and we don't want to add any more. If you are used to eating a lot of salt, this is a good time to cut back since a lot of salt will eventually make you very sick. High blood pressure, stroke, and all the rest come directly from excessive salt intake. Here's the good news. You will adjust to the lack of salt within a few days and you will then be able to detect and enjoy the natural salty flavor of the good food you are eating. In the meantime use lemon juice wherever you would have added salt before. You will be pleasantly surprised at the salty taste it produces.

2. *Vegetables.* This is good news for vegetable haters. For those of us who like vegetables, we won't miss them too much for a mere 7 days or 21 meals. In the meantime we are going to be so full and so contented that we won't worry about anything like that.

3. *No salt-preserved food.* That means we have to give up—*for one short week*—the following items:
   a. Sausage, ham, bacon, smoked or salted fish, and the like.
   b. Potato chips, corn chips. tortilla chips, etc.
   c. Pickles and relishes of all varieties—just because of their massive salt content.

4. *No bread.* That means no rolls, bread, buns, or the like. I promise you that you won't miss them. Wait and see.
5. *No pasta products.* That is, no spaghetti, no macaroni, lasagna, fettucini, noodles, etc.
6. *No candies, cakes, cookies, ice cream, or any other sweets.* You will be amazed that after about 2 hours on the diet you will suddenly lose any interest in these items.
7. *No rice, potatoes, or any other of the "starches".* Once again, you will be so full that you won't even think about these items.
8. *No alcoholic beverages*—with the very special exceptions that we will mention later on.

How do you put this all together to make interesting palatable meals? Very easy. Here are some typical menus that immediately come to mind. Once you get into it, I'm sure you can do much better.

BREAKFAST

1 cup of unsweetened yogurt with sliced apple on top
Cottage cheese—any amount
Tea or coffee with cream

LUNCH

Jumbo shrimp (as many as you like) fried in olive oil with garlic
Lettuce salad with oil and vinegar dressing
Tea or coffee with cream

DINNER

Sirloin steak (as much as you want)—leave all the fat on
Lettuce and tomato salad with mayonnaise
Tea or coffee with cream

Between meals, if you are really hungry, you can have as much cheese as you like—and I'd be happier if you'd spread a little mayonnaise on it at the same time. Try different varieties of cheese and you can also combine the cheese with other snack items on this diet. For example you can have a piece of chicken between two slices of cheese or a piece of cheese between two slices of chicken. Actually it's a good idea to eat six smaller meals rather than 3 larger ones so there's no need to feel guilty about eating in between regular mealtime. As we've said, this is a no-guilt, no-suffering diet. The only thing you have to lose is: excess weight. That's it. Plenty of good food, a lot of protein, a little extra fat and you will never be hungry for a moment.

Oh yes, there's one little point. The idea of *The Diet of Diets* is to lose weight promptly, painlessly, and pleasantly and with that in mind I always make special allowances for special tastes. If you are the kind of person who really misses fruit and vegetables in your diet, I can offer you a little escape hatch that will hardly make any difference at all in the final outcome—except you will lose weight a little slower. The fruit and vegetables that are included are very low in carbohydrate and will only slow you down a tiny bit.

Here are some more sample menus you can try for yourself:

BREAKFAST

3 slices of Swiss cheese garnished with three slices of tomato
Tea or coffee with cream

LUNCH

Deep fried fish with mayonnaise sauce—as much as you want
Lettuce salad with oil and vinegar dressing
Tea or coffee with cream

DINNER

Fried chicken (as much as you want)
Lettuce and tomato salad with mayonnaise
Tea or coffee with cream

At lunch and dinner you can also substitute nice things like half an avocado with mayonnaise, ¼ of a cantaloupe, 1 nectarine, 1 plum, 10 strawberries, or ½ cup of watermelon balls (or the equivalent amount of sliced watermelon) for the lettuce and tomato salad. It makes the module ever more enjoyable.

There's one other thing. I'm sure you may have noticed it. There aren't any alcoholic beverages in this module. But, I always have a pleasant surprise or two for you up my sleeve and this is no exception. It's really better not to drink when you're on a diet but if it's very important to you I've made room for one of the following at the end of each day *only if you have stayed on your diet one hundred per cent:*

> 1 ounce of whiskey
> 1 ounce of rum
> 1 ounce of vodka
> 1 ounce of gin

You can take it with water or soda—or straight if you like. But hold it to a bare ounce and use it as a reward if you've stuck to your diet 100% that day.

You say you don't drink liquor but you like a little wine? Fine. It's a bit trickier since the carbohydrate content of wine can vary from brand to brand. Make sure it is dry wine and buy the very best brand you can afford. That helps to assure us that there is no added sugar. Here's the list of wines to choose from:

> Dry Burgundy
> Dry Sherry
> Dry Sauterne
> Dry German white wines

The ration is 3 ounces once a day. As usual, only drink it as a reward when you have finished eating for the day and have followed your module to the letter.

Please bear in mind that your weight loss will be slower if you add liquor or wine to your diet. If you don't have a drink now and then will it drive you out of your mind? Well, I couldn't let that happen, could I?

There are two things about this module that I'm sure you noticed right away. First, there are no quantities specified. That's deliberate because you can eat as much as you want. If you want to eat a pound of cheese for breakfast, you can—although I doubt if you will ever try unless you are in a cheese-eating contest. You can have a cup or two cups of cottage cheese at breakfast—but you will probably want somewhat less. You can eat a dozen steaks if you care to—but I don't think you will.

The other little detail that I'm sure you observed is that the variety of foods is somewhat limited. There's a reason for that. At the beginning of this module I promised you that you would never feel hungry—and I delivered. But you have to trade freedom from hunger while you lose weight for an infinite variety of foods to choose from. The name of **Module One** is *The High Protein-Moderate Fate Anorexigenic Diet*. The key word there is: "anorexigenic". It's a bit of medical jargon that means: "takes your appetite away". And as you will see, it certainly does that. Very quickly you will get to the point where forcing yourself to eat lunch can be the hardest work you do all day. When it comes to dinner time, you may find it hard to wade even through a few mouthfuls of fish. But you should eat at least three meals a day— whether you are hungry or not. And sometimes we have to tolerate a bit of sameness in this module to work the miracle of "eat all you want and lose weight effortlessly".

There is one point worth emphasizing at this juncture. **Module One** gives you all the advantages of taking amphetamine diet pills with none of the risks. If you follow the instructions exactly it will abolish your appetite without clobbering your brain and without making you want to swing from the chandelier, punch the television set, or fly without wings. The way it helps you lose weight is magic. Well, almost magic. Like any other diet that works, **Module One** depends on a trick—a trick that is played on your digestive system and on your brain. It's a harmless trick and since we're going to do it for a very short period of time, it's doubly harmless. Since I don't ever keep any secrets from you, I'm going to tell you exactly what it does. This is it:

Protein has a very special effect on human beings that we take advantage of in **Module One**. It has what physiologists call "high satiety value". In plain English that means that a small amount of protein can go a long way to kill your appetite and keep you from getting hungry. Carbohydrates, on the other hand, fill you quickly, but in an hour or so, you're hungry again. The best example is the Chinese restaurant. Eat a lot of vegetables and plenty of white polished rice and you feel like bursting. But by the time you get home again, you're ready for another meal. However if you eat a good helping of roast beef for dinner, you may not get hungry until the next morning.

That's why **Module One** has a lot of protein in it and almost no carbohydrates. You eat cheese and fish and poultry in great abundance. As you eat this excellent quality diet, you benefit from the satiating effect of the protein. But the protein has to get well into the digestive system before it works its satisfying effect. That's the reason you have to eat slowly and if you should still be hungry, wait at least thirteen minutes before you take your second helping. But we do something else to make doubly sure that you won't be tempted to overeat.

We add a moderate amount of fat to **Module One**. Fat has an even greater satiating or satisfying effect than protein. When you eat something that is "rich" or high in fat content, you become full very quickly. That's the reason for frying everything and serving oil dressings and sauces as often as possible. The combination of high protein and a certain amount of fat gives a feeling of total satisfaction very quickly.

As if that were not enough, we work one more "magic" trick to assure your success. When we eliminate all or most carbohydrate from your diet, we change the way your liver processes the digested food. We shift the liver to a primarily protein and fat-oriented metabolism so that we encourage it to consume your body fat. In that way we hope to burn off whatever unwanted deposits of fat you may have around your body. Please notice that I say, "hope" because that's about where it is. No one really knows if we can get the liver to burn fat selectively although it would be nice. So let's just consider that possibility as an extra bonus if it works out that way.

I should probably mention at this point that you may run into someone who will tell you that **Module One** is hazardous to your health. You should ask them if being fat is good for your health. You can also point out that **Module One** is the typical diet of Inuits (formerly incorrectly called "Eskimos") and Indians who live in very severe climates as well as some African tribes who live under terribly harsh conditions. Ask the expert who tells you **Module One** isn't wonderful if he'd like to run a foot race across an ice floe with an Eskimo who has been on **Module One** all his life. Besides, the ancestors of those folks have been thriving on **Module One** for about 3 million years. I'm sure you can stay on it for a week without much trouble. In addition, these folks stay on **Module One** for a lifetime. We plan to follow it for a somewhat shorter period—168 hours or seven days.

Now we come to the final point for this module. What if we really like it and we're losing weight on it with almost no effort? Do we have to go on to the next module? It seems a shame to give up a diet we like and that's helping us lose weight. As with any other diet problem, we'll easily find the solution to that as well. We'll discuss it in detail farther on in the Chapter on "Diet Strategy". In the meantime, let's push on to some even more pleasant surprises in **Module Two**!

4

The Pleasure Principle And How To Enjoy

The Gratification Turning Point

Well, we're moving right along now, aren't we? I hope that you enjoyed **Module One**. I know that there's always a certain amount of anxiety when you start out on a new diet and I'm sure that **Module One** showed clearly that you don't have to suffer to be slim and healthy. There actually comes a point in your dieting experience where it becomes easier to stay on your diet than it is to deviate from it! That point is so crucial to your dieting success that I've given it a name. I call it "The Gratification Turning Point". For you and me there is nothing more important in dieting than the concept of "The Gratification Turning Point".

This is the way it works:

It's no secret to anyone who has been on a reducing diet that dieting is only really "fun" for a masochist. Even though I've gone to great lengths to make losing weight as painless as possible, with *The Diet of Diets* there is still some tiny remnant of deprivation involved. The fact is, we can't eat *everything* we want—that's how all this fat stuck to us in the first place. It's true that with *The Diet of Diets* we can eat as much as we want but we still have to be careful about our choice of food. And there is a long list of foods that we don't touch until we get down to our desired weight. In addition to all that, there are the *Four Fears* to contend with. *The Diet of Diets* zaps those four enemies of dieting success very nicely but they are always waiting to torment us in a weak moment—if we let them.

So losing weight is really a battle—a constant struggle—*A War!* Over the past four decades of treating overweight I've been fascinated to observe that there are some patients who win and some who lose. (Based on those observations, I designed *The Diet of Diets* in order to give everyone the greatest possible chance of winning.)

As I observed my patients, I discovered that there was a certain moment during their dieting experience when they suddenly had no trouble whatsoever following their diet. Almost overnight they were suddenly freed from all temptation, from all hesitation, and from all uncertainty. At what seemed to be a predetermined moment, they became "diet fanatics". From that point on, it would have taken a gun to their head—or worse—to make them eat something that was not going to help them achieve their goal. I began to investigate what really happened at the precise moment when each patient suddenly made the unconscious decision to make the diet he was on permanent and successful. What I discovered was interesting, fascinating, and useful to anyone who wants to be permanently thin and healthy.

I found that each patient had his own "magic moment"—a unique experience that happened suddenly and without warning. It was a moment of acute personal awareness that made a real difference in their future life. The best way is to let them describe it:

It happened to Jeanette like this:

"I'm 28 years old, Doctor, and I've always been heavy—which means 'fat'—ever since I can remember. And I've been dieting ever since I can remember. It was about 3 months ago that I started on *The Diet of Diets*. I weighed 155 pounds at the time and considering that I'm only 5 feet 3 inches tall, I was in trouble."

"Well, I'd been on *The Diet of Diets* for almost a week and I wasn't weighing myself every day like I should. The truth is, I was afraid to. I hadn't been hungry at all that entire week and although I followed the diet to the letter, I had been eating a lot—just like you recommended. I'd failed on every other diet I'd ever tried and I was afraid of failing again. So that morning—I'll never forget—it was a Saturday and I didn't have to go to work—I got up and finally decided to weigh myself. I'll admit, I was trembling. It seemed to me that if I couldn't succeed on *The Diet of Diets*, I was doomed to be fat forever."

"I stepped on the scale as lightly as I possibly could. First I put down my left foot. Then I closed my eyes because I was really scared. Then ever so lightly I dropped my right foot beside my left one. Then I opened one eye and peeked at the dial. I was down nine pounds! I couldn't believe it! It was the most wonderful thing that ever happened to me! From that moment on, I knew that I could finally be thin—once and for all. Now I'm down to 115 pounds and I'm on **Module Eight**—and loving every minute of it. And I'll never forget that Saturday morning as long as I live!"

For Jeanette, something clicked in her mind when she found that she could lose nine pounds swiftly and painlessly. At that precise moment she reached her own personal *gratification turning point*. The tremendous and lasting satisfaction she received from easily losing weight suddenly overwhelmed the puny pleasures of gorging herself on food she didn't need and usually hardly even enjoyed. For others, it happens in a different way. Let Paul tell it:

"I'm 43, Doctor, and I know I don't look it. That's the point. I'm chief teller in a big downtown bank and I have to deal with customers all day long. My appearance is often the first impression they get of the management of our bank. I used to weigh 195 pounds. I'm five feet seven and as you can see, I've lost some of my hair and it did make me look chubby and sort of, what shall I say, 'wimpy'? Well, you know what I mean."

Paul chuckled.

"Six months ago I started on *The Diet of Diets*—really in desperation. I couldn't get into any of my clothes and to be honest, I could hardly afford to buy a whole new wardrobe. So I went for the diet in a big way. In the space of a two months, I was down to 154 and I needed new clothes badly. I finally invested in a new suit but it was ..."

Paul stopped and blushed.

"What's the matter, Paul?"

"Well, it's a little embarrassing, Doctor. As I said, I wasn't making that much as chief teller and the only suit I could find at a reasonable price was something they had on sale and it wasn't what you'd expect in a bank. I mean, Elvis Presley used to wear more conservative clothes."

Paul shrugged his shoulders.

"It wasn't the kind of outfit I would have picked to wear to work but it was the only half-way decent suit they had in my size. It was pale-gray linen and pretty tight, if you now what I mean. Well, it actually made me look like maybe a skinny rock and roll musician on the way up—which when you come to think of it, is better than a fat chief teller on his way down …"

Paul grinned broadly as he continued.

"I'll tell you, Doctor, it really is a strange world. It wasn't a week later when the manager of our branch called me in. I thought he was going to chew me out for my weird taste in clothes. Instead, he told me I'd been promoted to Assistant Manager. You could have knocked me over with a feather! I was that surprised! But what surprised me even more was what he said."

"What was that?"

Paul chuckled.

"He said that the Board of Directors had decided to give the job to a younger man but they'd been watching me lately and it seemed to them that I was getting younger as each week went by! It turned out to be a lucky combination of the only suit I could afford and of course the 41 pounds I lost on *The Diet of Diets*. From that moment on, losing weight was no problem and now I'm finished at 129. And I can swear to you that I'll never gain another ounce. Oh yes, one more thing. With the first new paycheck, I went out and bought me a new suit—different color but the same material and the same style as my rock and roll model. That's what every up-and-coming Assistant Manager should wear!"

The experience may not be as dramatic for all of us as it was for Jeanette and Paul. For some of us it might happen this way:

You've been on *The Diet of Diets* about two weeks and you meet a friend on the street whom you haven't seen in a month or so. He blinks at you in amazement and says,

"What happened? You look great! What's your secret?"

Or you're a woman and you've been wearing one-piece bathing suits for at least ten years. Now that you're twenty pounds slimmer you try a basic bikini for your first summer week-end at the beach. For the first time in ten years you notice male heads snapping around when you walk by.

Or you're a salesman and suddenly you find that you have less trouble closing each sale and that you feel a sense of self-confidence and pride in your work that you didn't feel when you had thirty pounds of fat between you and your customers.

For everyone, it comes in a different way. But no matter how it comes, it's the big moment. It's the moment when we begin to collect abundant dividends from all the sacrifices that we made to lose weight. (Wait just a minute. We have to take that back. We didn't make *that* many sacrifices on *The Diet of Diets*.) Anyhow, the magic moment is the moment when we turn the corner and suddenly get more satisfaction from losing weight than we used to get from stuffing ourselves with all those fattening foods. We have re-discovered what psychologists call "The Pleasure Principle". We have stumbled, as it were, on the very useful and exciting technique of postponing immediate satisfaction for future gratification. Before we discovered *The Diet of Diets* most of us were literally slaves to our food. Whenever we found ourselves face-to-face with a piece of chocolate cake or a big plate of french fries or a sensational ice cream concoction, we were powerless to resist it. We pounced on it like a hungry cat on a juicy mouse, swallowed it in the fewest possible bites and as soon as it was safely in our stomach—we repented.

"Oh, I wish I hadn't eaten that!"

"Uhmmmm, that was so good! But I'll regret it tomorrow!"

"Delicious! But I know I'll hate myself in the morning!"

And when morning finally comes, we do hate ourselves. But by then it's too late to get that terribly fattening little morsel back on the plate. Isn't it strange how we completely forget how much harm overeating will do us until the moment that we are through overeating? It's as if we have a total temporary amnesia which completely obliterates any judgment or reasoning until we can wolf down that fattening mouthful. As soon as it hits our stomach, we repent—when it's too late.

Once we re-discover "The Pleasure Principle" things turn completely in our favor. We are instantly able to postpone the evanescent and fleeting pleasure of wolfing down a piece of pie and substitute the permanent and lasting pleasure of being thin, healthy, and attractive. Our re-discovery of "The Pleasure Principle" is even more significant than the original discovery that research psychologists made—for one important reason. Their awareness is "intellectual". That is, they came upon this concept by reasoning and logic. Their understanding is theoretical and superficial. They can talk about it and write about it and that sort of thing. Our awareness, on the other hand, is *emotional* We have felt it in the core of our being. It has suddenly struck us that being fat and unhealthy and unattractive has distorted our lives. That fat belly and those sagging thighs aren't worth all the spaghetti and candy and starches in the world! At the precise moment we recognize that fact, it's if someone slapped us in the face with a wet towel. It is as if we have stepped on a hot coal in our bare feet. It is as if we have jumped into an ice cold lake. We *know*, once and for all, that we can say *no*! and we will say *no*! to foods that make us fat and we will say *yes*! to a whole new look and a whole new life. Emotional awareness of the pleasure principle is what can make weight loss pleasant, permanent, and plausible. Once we go through that experience we are a different person. It is an emotional awareness that is almost mystical in its intensity. For those who experience it and understand it, overweight is a thing of the past—a bad dream that will never return to haunt them.

From that moment on, everything changes. We never "forget" to weigh ourselves in the morning. It's out of bed and onto the scale to see how much weight we have lost in the past 24 hours. Once we know what we're after, a simple and nutritious breakfast satisfies us completely. We go through the day without feelings of regret over the fattening snacks we have missed. We now find our satisfaction in our work and our personal relationships—not in potato chips and cheeseburgers. After dinner, we cannot be tempted by anything that will do us harm. And as we get closer and closer to our goal we get more and more satisfaction from our accomplishment. The gratification that we have been postponing—the gratification of a slim and healthy body—becomes ours even sooner then we expected.

With that in mind, let's move on to **Module Two**. **Module Two** is really exciting! It's a module that has been tested for about ten thousand years by about two billion people and it really works. There is no hunger, no sacrifice, no risk, and nothing but a smooth automatic weight loss. You're going to be surprised when you hear what it is. Let me present it to you and then I'll give you a detailed analysis of what you can expect from it. Here we go!

Module Two consists of three meals a day and all the meals have one thing in common, as we will see. Here it is:

BREAKFAST

Eight ounces of any fruit juice
4 ounces of any fruit
5 ounces of rice

LUNCH

Eight ounces of any fruit juice
4 ounces of any fruit
3 ounces of any vegetable
5 ounces of rice

DINNER

Eight ounces of any fruit juice
4 ounces of any fruit
3 ounces of any vegetable
5 ounces of rice

What am I trying to do? Do I want to turn America into a nation of Asiatics all bent meekly over rice bowls poking rice into their mouths with chopsticks? Hardly. What I want to do is save about one hundred million Americans from an early and unpleasant demise. This is the famous *Original Therapeutic Medical Rice Diet* designed in 1940 (not some later "popular" rice diet)—but adapted to *The Diet of Diets* so that it is pleasant and satisfying—extremely satisfying. First, let me tell you how it got started.

Quite a few years ago, doctors doing research into high blood pressure observed that high blood pressure as we know it is quite rare in Chinese and Japanese. Those are folks whose diets are primarily based on rice. As we all know, high blood pressure is a very serious problem. It kills tens of millions of people by producing heart attacks, heart failure, strokes, and other terrible and relentlessly fatal conditions. It cripples tens of millions of others and its actual cost in money terms is astronomical. Even today, with all the facilities of so-called "Modern Medicine", the treatment of high blood pressure is difficult. While there are very effective medicines that will bring down the blood pressure, they also tend to bring down other things. For example, one of the most effective medications also produces sexual impotence in men who take it. Other similar drugs cause mental depression and a bunch of awful side effects.

With that in mind, one of the researchers hit on the idea of asking his patients with severe high blood pressure to follow the Oriental diet. That is, a diet that is basically rice, fleshed out with fruit and vegetables. The one thing that had to be missing from the diet was that arch-enemy of good health: *Salt!* Salt isn't good for any of us but it is poison for those who suffer from high blood pressure or who may be susceptible to high blood pressure. Who is susceptible to high blood pressure? Well, everybody who eats too much salt, that's who.

Oh yes, I know. Salt is necessary. But you don't have to add a single grain of salt to the food that you eat—either before or after it is cooked—and you can stay perfectly healthy. As a matter of fact, you will be healthier than the people who shake salt onto everything. Here's the explanation:

Everything that you eat contains salt. Sodium and chloride are abundant in the soil of this planet and find their way into every animal and vegetable product that we consume. It is next to impossible to eat anything resembling a normal diet without getting adequate amounts of salt. Once you consume more than the minimum amounts of salt necessary for the functioning of your body, you are asking for trouble. And the truth is, most people are asking for trouble. Look at the facts:

The average person needs about 200 milligrams of salt a day to be healthy. That's about one twentieth of a teaspoonful—really not very much. The average person consumes about 3500 milligrams a day, approximately 4½ teaspoons! That's almost a full ounce of salt—*sixteen pounds* in one year—or one hundred times what we need to be healthy!

Where does all this salt come from and why? Most of the excessive salt in our diet comes from processed foods. Unfortunately when a natural food is canned, frozen, processed, or pasteurized, most of the taste goes out of it. In order to give it some kind of taste, the food processors add salt. Salt is cheap, convenient, and accepted by the great masses as a "flavor". The simple garden pea is a good example. If you eat fresh peas, they contain about 1 milligram of sodium per 100 grams. (Sodium content is the indicator for the amount of salt or sodium chloride in food.) If you choose canned peas, they have acquired 240 milligrams of sodium per 100 grams.

Somehow in the process of being canned, those little green peas have picked up a 239,000 per cent increase in salt content! What do you think that does to your blood pressure? ... not to mention your taste buds.

Almost everything that you buy in boxes, bottles, bags, cans, frozen or otherwise pre-prepared is loaded with salt. Here are some sample salt contents of popular foods:

Dried soup mixes: 2440 milligrams per serving
Bottled salad dressing: 600 milligrams per serving
Processed cheese: 500 milligrams per serving

The list goes on and on but the fascinating thing to note is that a *single serving* of any of these common products gives you about 500 per cent more sodium in a single day than you need or should have. Restaurant food is another example. Almost all the pizzas, hamburgers, fried chicken, fish and chips, and everything else you eat on the run is overdosed with salt to—how shall we put it? To make you less conscious of the real taste in the preparation and selection of the dish. A good slug of salt masks almost anything.

Now back to the rice. When the medical researchers placed patients with very severe high blood pressure on a rice diet, they were amazed at the results! Without any dangerous drugs the patients' blood pressure gradually fell to normal. The men and women on the diet reported a tremendous sense of euphoria and enthusiasm for life. Their general physical condition improved literally from one week to the next. But most important to us, *they all lost weight!*

These were people consuming over 2000 calories a day—a full pound of rice, plus fruit and vegetables in abundance—and they all lost weight! Based on those findings, I designed and adapted **Module Two** to make life easy for us. From a scientific and nutritional point of view, technically speaking, **Module Two** is: *The Carbohydrate Loading Anorexigenic Diet.* Translated back into English, that means, as always in *The Diet of Diets*, a diet that takes away all your hunger. That's the "anorexigenic" part. It also primes your liver and muscles with carbohydrate to give you tremendous amounts of energy. In this respect, it is similar to the diets that Olympic athletes consume just before their most difficult competitions. It increases their endurance, multiplies their motivation, and fortifies their capacity to win. I think that we will welcome all these benefits as we enter into the Weight Loss Olympics—a competition we are very interested in winning.

All right, now let's get down to business. It's best if you eat brown or unpolished rice rather than white rice for some obvious reasons. Unpolished rice has five times as much iron, five times as much vitamin B1 (thiamine) and twice as much niacin as the polished or white variety. It also has much more vegetable fiber—which is vitally important in any diet, reducing or otherwise. If you must eat "white" rice then please choose the "pre-cooked" or "par-boiled" or "converted" variety which keeps at least some of the original nutrients.

You can eat 5 ounces—*uncooked weight*—of rice three times a day or 2.5 ounces six times a day, for a total of one pound of cooked rice per day. That's a lot of rice. As a matter of fact, it's so much rice that you will never be hungry. You will also develop a feeling of energy and vitality that you have never had before. Don't take my word for it—just try **Module Two** for a few days and you'll see.

If you are using *brown* or *unpolished rice*, do it this way:

Put one pound of rice into a large pot and add enough cold water to cover the rice completely and about 1½ inches more. That is, the water should extend about 1½ inches above the top of the rice.

Put it on the highest heat, uncovered, until the water boils. Then reduce the heat to "low", cover, and leave for 45 minutes. Don't take the cover off to peek during this time. When the time is up, all the water should be evaporated and you should have a pot full of nice fluffy rice for the whole day. If you like your rice popped open or exploded, just leave it covered on low heat for about 10 or fifteen minutes longer. That's all there is to making perfect rice!

For *white* or *polished rice*, do it exactly the same way except leave it on low heat for only 20 minutes.

If you are going to use pre-cooked, parboiled, or "converted" rice, then simply follow the instructions on the label.

Some folks prefer to use those automatic electric rice-cookers. In that case, follow the instructions that come with the cooker.

Incidentally, since you know exactly how much rice you are going to consume at each meal, you may like the idea of cooking up five pounds or so at a time and then freezing it in individual 5 ounce plastic pouches. You can try it if you want to and see if you like it.

If you're not going to cook your rice fresh for each meal, then you will be heating it up again. One of the easiest ways to do that is to put the rice in a frying pan, sprinkle it with water to moisten it well, cover it, and place on low heat. Stir it from time to time, and you should quickly have a nice steaming portion of delicious rice.

We were just speaking about vitamins and I don't want you to worry about vitamin deficiencies under any circumstances. All the menus in *The Diet of Diets* will provide you with every possible vitamin and mineral you might need. Really. So you don't have to worry about that—ever.

The one thing that you can't have any of on this module is: salt. But don't worry. Even if you've been a salt glutton up until now, after a few days without gobs of salt in everything, you will begin to taste the natural salt in your food—including the rice—and you will discover a whole new world of flavor. Extra salt tends to overwhelm any of the natural flavors and aromas in your food and when you cut back on it, everything begins to take on a superb taste and aroma that was never there before. You'll see what I mean once you get started. In addition, I'll tell you a trick or two that will give you the flavor of salt without the damage. By the way, the rules against salt also include a chemical called "monosodium glutamate", otherwise known as "MSG" and sold under may different trade names. MSG is widely used to perk up the flavor of over-processed and de-nutrified foods. It contains a lot of sodium and can be as bad for high blood pressure as salt. Now let's take a look at some sample menus:

BREAKFAST

8 ounces of orange juice
One medium size sliced banana
5 ounces rice
Tea or coffee without milk, cream, or sugar

In this case, you can eat the rice as you would a breakfast cereal, with the fruit on top. I should also mention that you will probably prefer tea rather than coffee with **Module Two** but you may have either.

LUNCH

8 ounces apple juice
4 ounces of melon
1½ ounces of cooked mushrooms and 1½ ounces of cooked peas
5 ounces of rice
Tea or coffee without milk, cream, or sugar

DINNER

8 ounces of grape juice
4 ounces of red raspberries
1½ ounces of cooked onions and 1½ ounces of cooked green pepper
5 ounces of rice
Tea or coffee without milk, cream, or sugar

For both lunch and dinner, you should mix your rice with the vegetables and enjoy a rather nice dish. You can use pepper or horseradish or any other natural spice or seasoning—but no commercial seasonings, and of course, no soy sauce.

Here's another important point to watch. Ideally all the fruits, fruit juices, and vegetables you use should be fresh. They have much more nutritional value that way and they certainly taste better. But if you absolutely have to, you can use frozen fruits, fruit juices, or frozen vegetables instead. However you must be perfectly sure that they don't have any added salt or sugar. You should avoid canned fruits, canned fruit juices, and canned vegetables since they are nutritionally inferior and it's hard to be sure that they don't have sugar and salt dumped into them. That's the other problem. Without added sugar and salt, canned foods are tasteless and drag down the whole appeal of **Module Two**. So hold out for fresh fruits, fruit juices, and vegetables. It's worth the effort.

Considering that you are eating rice, you may want to try some of the many varieties of Chinese and Japanese teas as an accompaniment. It will make your diet that much more interesting.

That brings up another question: What do you do at work? Do you shuffle in with your rice bowl and chop sticks? Hardly. If you are in the habit of eating lunch at a restaurant, you can simply choose from one of the many Chinese, Japanese, Thai, Viet Nam, Cambodian, Burmese, or other Oriental restaurants. Order a big serving of boiled rice and ask them to prepare it without salt—or monosodium glutamate—and have them add the unsalted vegetables you prefer. You will find a very warm reception at almost any Oriental restaurant with such a request since that's the way many Orientals take their rice.

If you want to take your lunch along with you, you can simply prepare it before you leave and pop the rice into one of those wide-mouthed thermally-insulated plastic containers and it will be piping hot when lunch time rolls around. You can also try some nice cold rice.

Please don't wrinkle up your nose like that. It's not just any old cold rice. It's the elegant and traditional Japanese dish known as "sushi"—you just might fall in love with it. Here's a modified version for **Module Two**:

Divide your 5 ounces of cold cooked rice into 6 or 8 individual patties. Add a bit of vinegar—according to your taste—to each patty. You can select the type of vinegar you prefer but make sure it is pure vinegar—without salt or other unknown ingredients.

On top of each patty place one or more of the following:

Cold thinly-sliced cucumber
Cold thinly-sliced mushrooms
Cold thinly-sliced watercress
Cold thinly-sliced fresh pineapple
… or thin slices of any fresh fruit or vegetable that you prefer.

You can then sprinkle it with ground ginger, horseradish, lemon juice or any other natural spice you desire. Incidentally, if you really miss salt at the beginning of the diet, you can squeeze liberal amounts of fresh lemon juice over your meals. For many people—in the days before their taste buds adjust to the reduction of excess salt, it provides just the "salty" flavor that they are looking for. Try sushi—you might like it.

So with the ability to eat the rice cold or hot and to combine it with any unsalted fruit or vegetable, **Module Two** becomes a diet of infinite variety and very wide-appeal. And remember, don't waste a moment worrying about vitamins or minerals. Just to make sure you don't worry, let's do a nutritional analysis of a typical lunch. Here we go:

Grape Juice: Contains essential vitamins and minerals except vitamin A.

Red Raspberries: Contains essential vitamins and minerals plus generous amounts of vitamin A.

Onions: Contains essential vitamins and minerals.

Green Pepper: Contains essential vitamins and minerals.

Rice: Contains every essential vitamins and minerals except vitamin C. The raspberries, green peppers, and onions contain substantial amounts of vitamin C. The rice provides about 4 grams of protein per meal.

Even this very simple meal is nutritionally complete and far better balanced than the vast majority of reducing diet menus. Considering that **Module Two** is only planned for 21 consecutive meals, there is no risk whatsoever. And there is virtually a guarantee that we will find ourselves thinner and happier at the end of the week. We will also be the beneficiaries of several other fringe benefits of **Module Two**:

1. We will never be hungry on this module—not for an instant.
2. We will probably lower our blood pressure if it is high and protect ourselves from high blood pressure if our pressure is normal.
3. We will have plenty of energy and zip—more than when we began **Module Two**.
4. We will never run the risk of becoming wrinkled or scrawny on **Module Two**—or any of the other modules of *The Diet of Diets*.

With that in mind, let's not waste any more time. Get out the rice and let's get started on an exciting and rewarding week on **Module Two**!

5

Now Let's Have Some Fun!

Now we're getting to a module that's really fun! **Module Three** amazes everyone. It seems so simple and so easy but what it does for weight loss is nothing less than spectacular!

It has some other superb advantages as well. For anyone who has to eat at work, for someone who travels a lot, for dieters who are away at school, for people who keep irregular hours, **Module Three** is made to order. It is the simplest, most portable of all modules and yet it is among the most satisfying. You can carry it with you or buy it inexpensively almost anywhere. Yet for all its simplicity, it is totally satisfying and perfectly balanced nutritionally—like all the modules on *The Diet of Diets*. And of course, you can eat as much as you want on **Module Three**, just like any module on *The Diet of Diets*.

But **Module Three** requires something extra of us, if we are going to be able to get the most of it. It requires a tiny bit more experience in dieting than the first two modules. That's why we presented **Module One** and **Module Two** first. Of course, let's keep in mind that our Master Dieting Strategy may recommend that we begin with **Module Three** or perhaps even **Module Seven**, but we'll explore that in detail farther along in our dieting program.

Let's take a moment now to think about what "experience" in dieting means. Like almost any other skill—tennis, golf, billiards— dieting can be "learned". Just a minute—how do you learn *not* to eat?

Well, dieting is more than just not eating just as tennis, golf and billiards are much more than just smacking the ball. You can diet as a beginner or do it as a professional. One of the outstanding characteristics of the sophisticated dieter is his attention to details.

For example, he is careful to put what he expects to eat at that sitting on his plate all at once—so that the only food before him is what he is reasonably going to consume. That means, say, a leg and a breast of chicken and a small container of *hollandaise* sauce if he is on **Module One** or 5 ounces of rice with his choice of fruit and vegetables if he is on **Module Two**. That's a small detail but it avoids the unnecessary temptation of your plate overflowing with steaming goodies sitting there just begging to be eaten.

Yes, I know, on *The Diet of Diets* we can eat as much as we want but it's common sense to make life as easy as possible for ourselves in the process. For example, if we are going to give up smoking, we don't surround ourselves with packets of cigarettes, elegant ashtrays, and posters of beautiful people smoking in luxurious surroundings. Oh yes, that's something else. Don't watch television or read magazines while you eat or within half an hour before eating. Sound strange? Not really. Think about how many programs and commercials on TV show people eating delicious food in exciting surroundings. Think about how many advertisements in magazines show appetizing food and people enjoying it.

This is just the kind of powerful emotional stimulation that we are trying to avoid. One of the basic strategies of *The Diet of Diets* is to change the roles that food plays in our lives. What roles does food play in our lives? For those of us who are overweight, food plays many roles. It is a tranquilizer, a consolation, an entertainment, a defense mechanism, a barrier against the world, a status symbol, a reward, revenge, sexual satisfaction, masochism, sadism, and about fifty other things except what it really is: a source of nourishment to keep our minds and bodies functioning in a normal and healthy way.

Secondarily, of course, food can be a source of sensual pleasure. You know, a bowl of soup warming us on a chilly day, a nice steamed lobster, a slice of fresh-from-the-oven bread generously spread with newly-churned butter—and endless other examples that most of us can think of when we get hungry.

Speaking about hungry, did you ever stop to think what "hunger" really means? Most of us are the unwilling puppets of our own feelings of hunger. As we go through the day, at certain moments we suddenly have a funny feeling in our tummies that makes us panic and eat about three times as much as we really need. Then the feeling goes away for a few hours and we wait for it to come back again. Very often we eat even though we don't have that feeling. On the other hand, we hardly ever let that funny tummy sensation strike us without eating. When you start to think about it, it seems a little strange doesn't it? It gets even stranger when you study it a little further and realize that hardly anyone really understands exactly what "hunger" is. Those funny feelings that we call "hunger" come from two primary sources. Once we understand these sources we can put the knowledge to good use to make our weight loss program even more successful.

The most immediate sensation of hunger comes from physical contractions of the stomach wall. In the average person, about every five hours, the level of sugar (or glucose) in the blood begins to fall. That's because in the course of our usual activities, we consume our most readily-available carbohydrate stores. When our blood sugar drops, the muscles in the walls of our stomach begin to contract and we feel it as a vague sensation of discomfort. It's almost like someone tugging at our sleeve to attract our attention. If we ignore the signals, the tugging becomes more and more insistent. But just like someone tugging at our sleeve, it we continue to ignore it, it eventually goes away. That's the first important point to remember when we are dealing with hunger. People who fast—who go days or weeks without eating anything at all—lose all feelings of hunger within a day or so.

What does that mean to those of us who are on a diet? Well, it means good news because we don't have to be afraid of being hungry. It isn't going to kill us, it isn't going to harm us, and as a matter of fact, it will very quickly go away. Of course if you are on the *The Diet of Diets* you don't have to worry since you are never going to be hungry—not for one moment. But certainly we will feel better while dieting if we lose all fear of hunger in the process.

The next fact about hunger is just as interesting. Even if the blood sugar level is maintained at normal values, people get "hungry" every five hours or so. That part of hunger depends on conditioned reflex and habit. We are used to getting a little restless when noon rolls around. We welcome the change of scene and the relaxation that goes along with lunch time. After a hard day, when darkness falls, we look forward to sitting down to a nice meal and having a little fun. If we should forget, our tummy is there to churn a bit and remind us.

But sometimes, even if we have eaten recently—say within a couple of hours—we can still get hungry if we smell a favorite dish being cooked or see something we like being eaten on television or in a movie. That emotionally-determined "hunger" is completely independent of both blood sugar levels and conditioned reflexes.

If we understand and remember these three primary rules of hunger, we can use that knowledge to help ourselves lose weight quickly and easily on *The Diet of Diets*:

1. Feelings of hunger go away if you don't pay attention to them.
2. A big part of hunger is based on a conditioned reflex—the expectation of eating once every five hours or so.
3. Hunger can seize us as a result of seeing or smelling appetizing food—even if we have normal blood sugar levels and have eaten relatively recently.

If we stop to think about it, we will realize that most of what we think of as "hunger" is really nothing more than a desire for food—a certain craving based on the wish to consume something especially appetizing. The truth is that in this over-fed nation of ours, very few people have ever really felt hunger. If you are ever in doubt the way to tell the difference is this:

If you are hungry you will eat anything.

If you are merely feeling your appetite, you want to eat something specific.

As they used to say, if you're desperately hungry, a scrap of moldy bread will do fine. So if you think that unbearable hunger is a big obstacle to losing weight, just ask yourself how many moldy scraps of bread you've eaten this week …

Now let's take a moment to consider some of the other non-nutritional roles that food plays in our lives and whether it makes sense to use it that way—or allow it to use us that way. Here are a few of the most common non-food uses of food:

1. TRANQUILIZER

How many times in our lives when we have been tense or nervous or upset have we reached for something to pop into our mouth? When the going gets tough, how often do we start gobbling everything in sight? When was the last time we met adversity by stuffing ourselves horribly? Of course, we don't do that. But I bet we know some people who do …

When you're feeling bad, when things aren't going right for you, when all the world seems to be going in the opposite direction from you, that's the time when gorging yourself seems to be the only way out. Have you ever stopped to think what kind of food is the most "gorge-able"? Why, sweets, of course. Cookies, candy bars, cake, pie, tea or coffee with massive amounts of sugar, ice cream, puddings—this is the menu of tranquilization. But why? Because when things went wrong for baby, it was a good swig of mother's milk or overly-sweet baby formula. That therapy was so deeply-engraved in our minds that it will never be erased. Now grown-up babies don't reach for a nursing bottle when the going gets rough. But they do reach for the closest substitute: sweets and sugar, in any form.

What's wrong with that? Just this. Imagine that you are walking down a dimly-lighted street in some big city at midnight. Suddenly from a doorway, a thug leaps out and grabs you around the neck, twisting hard. In a panic, you summon up all your strength and deliver a powerful punch—*right to your own nose*!

That's the problem with food as a "tranquilizer". It does all the wrong things to you at all the wrong times. If you are having trouble with your husband or wife, making yourself fat isn't going to make your problem easier. If you have trouble at work, putting on pounds isn't going to make you more desirable as an employee. If you don't have the kind of social life you're wishing for, fifteen more pounds isn't going to perk up your social calendar. The real irony is this:

Food is not a tranquilizer. In fact it is and anti-tranquilizer.

Whatever problems you may have in life are made worse, much worse, by overeating. If you can only remember that, your goal of weight reduction will be so much easier to achieve.

2. STATUS SYMBOL

Some people might say, "Tell me what you eat, and I will tell you who you are." That concept has led millions of otherwise rational men and women to pay extravagant prices for eggs from a rather turgid fish that swims in certain territorial waters of Persia. It also maintains astronomical prices for nests of certain cliff birds in South-East Asia and keeps the price of dorsal fins of some elasmobranch species close to the international price of pearls.

Why else should people undergo great sacrifices for the privilege of consuming caviar, birds' nest soup, and shark fins? Why else should the price of less-nutritious cuts of meat be in the stratosphere while the more nutritious cuts often go into dog food? How often have you chosen liver, brains, sweetbreads (pancreas and thymus gland), and kidney over prime rib and T-Bone steak—when someone else was buying the dinner? You are eating plain old muscle from the cow when the organs contain all the wonderful nutrients.

When food becomes a status symbol it suddenly becomes a threat to our well-being—and not just our financial well-being. Since it costs so much and has acquired such an important emotional value, we eat it whether we are hungry or not and whether we really feel like eating.

That's what puts the pounds on faster than the blink of an eye. Expensive and fattening food may be a status symbol but a fat belly, a heart attack, or a chronic case of diabetes is strictly downscale in any social circle. It makes sense to eat to nourish our bodies. It can make sense to eat to enjoy our food. But it never makes sense to eat to impress the people around us …

3. REWARD

The mistaken use of food as a reward is probably the fault of some long-forgotten uncle or aunt. When we were good little girls or boys instead of giving us a dollar they slipped us a chocolate bar or a few cookies. It also goes back to those birthday parties when our reward for merely growing another year was an orgy of overly-frosted sickly-sweet birthday cake, sugary soda pop, mountains of sweet-and-fatty ice cream and cookies and candy that went on forever. A similar ceremony was repeated at graduations, weddings, anniversaries, and on and on. The dubious privilege of consuming immense amounts of fattening food was engraved on our minds as the reward for almost any accomplishment.

A thousand years ago in the days of half-civilized and half-starving tribes, a great celebration with conspicuous wastage of the tribe's limited food supply was an important ceremonial occasion. But in modern day America gorging ourselves with the excuse of a wedding anniversary is at best a negative reward. It would be far more appropriate to eat only the most healthful and simple meal on that occasion in order to make sure that we are alive and in good health for the next anniversary to come. I know, no one does it that way. But once we understand the symbolism and the hazards of "reward eating", we can enjoy the occasion without going overboard and turning a momentary pleasure into an extended regret.

4. SADO-MASOCHISM

Hold on just a moment! Am I trying to tell you that food can be an instrument of sado-masochism? Yes, that's exactly what I am telling you. First, let's define "sado-masochism". It's enjoying pain as a pastime. Sadists are keen on making other people suffer and masochists get their kicks from suffering. That leads to the old joke that the definition of sadism is "… being kind to a masochist". Maybe. But in the real world, sadism and masochism often occur simultaneously in the same person and the whole little drama can be acted out at the dinner table. Now I'm not trying to tell you that some folks get their jollies from being whipped with a stalk of asparagus or tickled with a bunch of parsley. But ask yourself this question:

"How many times have I eaten something that I really didn't enjoy with the acute awareness that I was going to regret it later on?" If you can remember a single occasion, that's an example of gastronomic masochism. You don't have to be a Professor of Psychiatry to recognize that as a distortion of eating. The purpose of food is to nourish your body, not to punish it. If you are ever eating anything and in the process of chewing it, you get the feeling that you are going to hate yourself in the morning, *stop!*—then and there. Don't make yourself the masochistic victim of a pizza or a taco. It really isn't worth it …

The sadistic part of eating is a bit more subtle. Very often it takes the form of an indulgent and well-meaning hostess who insists:

"Oh you simply must have another serving of my very special rum cake with whipped cream and chocolate curls!"

Does that sound as if she is just being hospitable? If you think so, try refusing politely. Her next assault will be something like this:

(Pronounced with a mock frown and mock irritation in the voice)

"I'm going to be ever so angry if you don't take another piece. You know, it's really my specialty!"

Your hostess knows that bulge around your waistline isn't going to get any smaller with yet another helping of her rum cake. And still she insists again—with a thinly-veiled but clearly recognizable threat behind her generosity. If she happens to be married to the president of the company you work for, you are going to be compelled to eat as many pieces of rum-and-chocolate cake as she wants to sadistically inflict upon you.

What's the defense against nutritional sadism? There's only one that's really effective—and at the same time, socially acceptable. It's this:

Hostess: (Making a pretend-angry face)

"Now I'm going to get terribly put-out if you turn down another helping of my stuffed pork chops. You know, they're famous all over the state."

Us: (Fighting back the urge to ask exactly what the pork chops are famous for, we spasmodically clutch some vague area of our chest and grunt ...) "Oh, I almost forgot! It's time to take my heart pills and I should have taken them on an *empty stomach*! I hope it's going to be all right!"

Only the most hardened dinner table sadist can stand up to that one ...

Now I'm afraid that you're going to start accusing me of nutritional sadism if I don't begin to tell you all about **Module Three**. I certainly wouldn't want that to happen, so here:

Module Three occupies a very special place in *The Diet of Diets*. Although it may not be the kind of module that you would like to stay with for the rest of your life, it is very satisfying, very nourishing, and nutritionally it is excellent. Here's the way it shapes up from the standpoint of protein, vitamins, minerals, and fiber:

Protein: A whopping 53 grams of protein per day!

Fat: Barely 2 grams, qualifying as a low fat diet.

Carbohydrate: 208 grams, which is quite adequate.

Plus very generous amounts of calcium, iron, phosphorus, copper, Vitamin A, Vitamin B1, Vitamin B2, Vitamin B6, Vitamin B12, Vitamin C, Vitamin E, and Vitamin K.

It will also give you as much as you need of niacin, pantothenic acid, and folic acid. As a bonus, it also contains quite a bit of dietary fiber.

It is a module that you could live on indefinitely and grow happier and healthier—and progressively thinner. It will banish your hunger completely and you will grow fonder of it as each day passes.

But before we get to that, it's important to put it in perspective.

If you really want to lose weight swiftly and safely, you have to be bold and inventive. In **Module Three**, we are taking all our knowledge of metabolism and nutrition and crafting a 21 meal program to turbocharge your weight-loss success.

Ready for a pleasant surprise? Here it is:

MODULE THREE

Breakfast: 1 raw banana

Second Meal: (exactly one hour later) 1 glass of skimmed milk

Third Meal: (exactly one hour later) 1 raw banana

Fourth Meal: (exactly one hour later) 1 glass of skimmed milk

Fifth Meal: (exactly one hour later) 1 raw banana

Sixth Meal: (exactly one hour later) 1 glass of skimmed milk

Seventh Meal: (exactly one hour later) 1 raw banana

Eighth Meal: (exactly one hour later) 1 glass of skimmed milk

Ninth Meal: (exactly one hour later) 1 raw banana

Tenth Meal: (exactly one hour later) 1 glass of skimmed milk

Fascinating, isn't it? You really have to try it to realize how simple and elegant and satisfying this diet is. It provides a perfect response to *fear of being hungry* since you are never more than 59 minutes away from your next meal. In addition you are eating ten meals a day – and still losing weight! No other diet in history can make that offer!

You can find what you need almost anywhere in this great country of ours or take it along with you wherever you go. A full day's ration is five bananas and about a liter of skimmed milk. If you feel you might have any difficulty getting the milk, you can simply take along little envelopes of instant powdered skimmed milk and mix it with water— and there you are! Of course, you can have as much tea or coffee as you like without cream or sugar but with a bit of milk. A little additional milk won't do you any harm.

Remember, as in all the other modules, only eat when you are hungry. If you don't want all ten items in the module, you don't have to eat them. If you prefer to space them farther apart, you can do that as well. But you shouldn't eat anything except the skimmed milk and the bananas. You will be amazed at how quickly and easily your weight will drop in the course of seven days on **Module Three**. Try it—you'll like it!

6

It All Starts In The High Chair

"Among the grimmest and most terrible tales are those which are told by the bathroom scales ..."

Only those who have been really overweight can testify to the truth of the preceding lines. Being fat is a very special form of martyrdom which must be suffered in silence and endured in frustration.

Someone who has never been fat at some time in their lives can't even imagine what it is to be really overweight. The pain and the deprivation is so great that fat people have developed a special "folklore of fatness" to rationalize their handicap. I'm sure you've heard it many times:

"Of course, I wish I could slim down but there's no chance. Overweight runs in my family. Everyone on both sides is heavy. My father weighed 200 pounds and my mother only a bit less. You can't argue with the genes now, can you?"

What's missing from this little narrative is the fact that Father ate enough for three men and died from a heart attack at the age of 54. Mother hardly ate at meals, preferring to stoke up in the kitchen when no one was watching. She lingered on a few years more until her organism finally succumbed to the massive doses of sugar she was constantly forcing upon it.

Some fat people are more direct:

"I don't know, I just feel better when I'm heavy. If I start losing weight I'm fine for the first week or so and then I get depressed and irritable. I suppose you might say being fat is the price I pay for staying on an even keel emotionally."

Occasionally someone says the same thing in a different way:

"Well, you do have to admit that fat folks are jollier!" (This declaration is almost always punctuated by a hearty Santa Claus-type laugh)

"Well, we are! You can't deny that we're friendlier and easier to get along with than you skinny guys!"

Maybe. But could it be that fat folks have to be friendly with everyone because if things turn ugly, they can't run away?

Perhaps not. But there is obviously a profound psychological basis for persistent overweight. One of the most important clues can be found in the cases of the individuals who get depressed when they begin to thin down. People who are persistently and significantly overweight have one very important characteristic in common: they want to "get".

Think about it this way: those people who are fat are fat for one very special reason. They are fat because they eat more than they need to eat to maintain their bodies in optimum condition. Sounds too simple, doesn't it? No, it doesn't sound simple at all when you ask the next question.

Why do they eat more than they need to eat to supply their physical needs? All we have to do is keep following that line of reasoning and we come smack up against a fascinating discovery.

Overweight people are eating to satisfy a need that goes beyond a *physical* need. They eat to satisfy an *emotional* need. I know what you're thinking. You're thinking that that's probably not an earth-shaking revelation—everyone assumes that fat people over-eat to satisfy an emotional hunger. I couldn't agree more. But hang on—there's another question about to emerge—and along with another answer. And that answer does qualify as "earth-shaking".

Here's the question: How in the world can stuffing one's tummy with food that one doesn't need satisfy an emotional need? I mean, is the digestive system directly connected to the brain? Why should a big dish of ice cream or a massive helping of chocolate cake make someone feel better? How can three helpings of pizza possibly improve someone's mood? Those are interesting questions, aren't they? Here are some interesting answers:

Although we may not think of it that way, food is emotion. Food is love. Food is security. Food is ten per cent nutrition and ninety per cent satisfaction. If it weren't that way, we would all be happy to eat the same perfectly balanced diet every day of our lives. Breakfast, lunch, and supper would be identical and all the restaurants in the country would be designed like post offices. Step up to the window, order your standard lunch ration, have your credit card punched, and make way for the next person. As we all know, it will never be that way. Every restaurant is a stage set complete with a mythology, a fantasy, a set of costumed performers, and even a cast of customers.

From the simplest fast food emporium to the fanciest pseudo-French bistro, food stands aside as fantasy occupies center stage. But why is it that way? Well, here's the answer and I hope you're ready for it. The dramatic value of food originates with the first and most exciting drama of them all: mother and child.

From an infant's first moments in this world, his life revolves around food and mother. When he is hungry, his mother is there with milk. Warm, sweet, fresh, nourishing milk. At the same time he gets the milk, he gets love. His mother picks him up, cuddles him, talks to him softly, sings to him and fills his little heart with love at the same time she fills his little stomach with food. (At least that's the way it's supposed to be.)

This unique and delightful experience is repeated approximately four to six times a day in the early months and at least three times a day for the rest of babyhood. In the beginning, feeding time is the principal moment of contact with the outside world. The baby sleeps and eats—that's that. Later on, it is the primary moment of gratification during his baby-day. The impressions that are engraved on the infant's conscious and unconscious mind during those early formative years are indelible impressions that influence his attitudes, reactions, and psychological choices for the rest of his life. In that set of early experiences, there is material for several sets of encyclopedias of human behavior. But to you and me who are sharing this adventurous journey through the uncharted wasteland of weight reduction, it's the link between baby feeding and adult overfeeding that interests us the most.

As a child gets older, more and more gratifications enter his life. There is the pleasure of accomplishment, of physical activity, the excitement of learning about a whole new universe that surrounds him. Little by little, the gratification of eating is replaced by the gratification of being part of the exciting world of human beings. Not entirely replaced, mind you, because food and sex are permanent instincts imprinted on every living species of animal—including the human ones. But every new satisfaction in life crowds out a certain percentage of gratification in eating. If a month old baby gets 90% of his emotional satisfaction from eating, we would expect an adult to get much less. Let's look at a couple of interesting examples:

Jane is twenty-four years old and about to be married. She is five feet four inches tall and weighs 116 pounds. She has long black hair that falls gently over her shoulders and her dark eyes glisten as she talks:

"I can't believe how exciting it all is! I mean between getting ready for the wedding in a month, doing my work as an art instructor, and spending every evening with Bob, my fiancé, I barely have time to eat, much less develop an appetite! Oh, I do eat three meals a day but sometimes by evening, I don't even remember what I had for lunch!"

In Jane's case, food probably only supplies a bare ten per cent of her emotional satisfaction. Now let's look at Bob, her fiancé.

Bob is a thirty year old Regional Sales Manager for an electronics company who is working hard at climbing the corporate ladder. He puts in long hard hours motivating his salesmen and calling on customers. But let him tell about it. Bob is tall and slim—at six feet he weighs 160 pounds.

"Jane's always chiding me about being too thin but to tell you the truth, I scarcely think about eating."

Bob grinned.

"However, I do think a lot about Jane. And between her and my work, eating seems so unimportant. I have a good chance to be named National Sales Manager next year and maybe then I'll be able to sit down and have some relaxed meals."

As things are now, Bob probably gets even less than 10% of his gratification in life from food. But let's jump in the Time Machine to leap ahead to the future and look at Bob and Jane ten years from now.

Unfortunately, Bob hasn't made it any farther up the corporate ladder. As a matter of fact he's slipped down a rung or two. His firm fell on hard times and he had a personal conflict with one of the owners. Eventually he was demoted to ordinary salesman. Now at the age of forty he feels he has little future in the business world. His relationship with Jane has suffered as a result and life between them is full of tension. Would it surprise you to discover that Bob now weighs in at 244 pounds? Eating is virtually his only satisfaction in life. And he does it with a vengeance. Listen to his description:

"You know, it used to be I had to be reminded to eat. I'd sometimes skip lunch because I was so busy. Now at 10 o'clock I find myself glancing at the clock to see when I can leave my desk and pop over to the snack bar and have a little snack."

Bob smiled sheepishly.

"Well, maybe more than just a little snack. You know, a couple of sandwiches—say, some ham and cheese on rye and a bag or two of potato chips. After all, a man gets hungry ..."

He rolled his eyes and patted his more than ample stomach.

Back home, Jane stroked a few wisps of hair away from her eyes. She had the same bright eyes but somehow they seemed smaller—lost in the immensity of her face with its three chins. She laughed nervously.

"I know what you're thinking. What happened to me? Well, it came on so gradually. I mean, Bob had that trouble at work and he always came home so out of sorts. You know, our sex life just evaporated after awhile and then there were money problems and the children. It seems that the only thing left was a good meal once in a while. I mean, I'm going to start losing weight as soon as the children go back to school. After all, I'm only up to 146 pounds and it shouldn't take me too long to get down to where I belong."

Jane smiled and smoothed her skirt down over her ample hips.

"By the way, I was about to have some coffee. I have some wonderful cookies just coming out of the oven. Would you care to join me?"

The love and affection that a twenty-four year old woman doesn't get from drinking her baby-milk she can get from her husband and her children. But if she doesn't get gratification from them—or from anywhere else—she has to get it from chocolate chip cookies ... and french fries and hamburgers and chocolate sundaes and orange soda—and—well, you know the rest.

If Bob can find satisfaction in achieving his goals in the world of business and finding happiness with his wife and children, then food can never eclipse the real satisfactions in his life. But if there is nothing else—no love, no sex, no accomplishment—then there is at least the sensual and psychological pleasure of stuffing himself with hot coffee loaded with cream and sugar and ham-and-cheese-on-rye.

Now this is a diet book, not a book on overcoming emotional problems. (For emotional problems, may I suggest a book entitled, *Dr. David Reuben's Mental First-Aid Manual—Instant Relief! ... from 23 of life's worst problems?*) But if we are going to be successful in losing weight we must at least have a working knowledge of the emotional factors that can cause us trouble. So, it makes sense to set our emotional house in order as much as we possibly can as we benefit from the unique advantages of *The Diet of Diets*.

Now let's move ahead to **Module Four**. After all the experience we've had with the first three modules, **Module Four** is going to be a piece of cake. Well, not exactly a piece of cake—better said, a piece of *protein*. Because **Module Four** is the outstanding example of the rational and scientific use of protein in weight reduction. Remember when we analyzed the various steps that food goes through in the process of digestion? Remember the fascinating relationships we discovered between the three major categories of food—protein, carbohydrate, and fat? Well, we're going to go one step further now and use a very special trick of digestive metabolism to produce a superb and effortless weight loss in the next twenty-one meals.

Let's review for a moment the results of oxidizing the different types of foods in the famous "bomb" calorimeter—that little chamber where food components are burned and the amount of heat given off is measured. Protein yields 5,300 calories for each gram that is burned in the experimental chamber. But when an equal gram of protein is burned—that is digested—in the human body, only 4,100 calories are produced! That means that somewhere, somehow, 1,200 calories are lost forever! For anyone who wants to lose weight, that is sensational news! It means that they can eat exactly the same amount of food and take in at least 25% fewer calories! All they have to do is eat only protein instead of a combination of fat, protein, and carbohydrate. But what happens to the other 25% of the calories? Interesting question. Here are some equally interesting answers:

1. We know that the metabolism of protein in the human body is notoriously inefficient. Instead of converting protein directly to energy, there are many intermediate steps that waste the energy which otherwise might be available for the body's needs. If you are shipwrecked on a desert island in the midst of a vast ocean, that's bad news. If you are metabolically shipwrecked in the midst of a vast ocean of fat, that's the best news you could ever hear.

2. Fat and carbohydrate cannot be converted to protein but protein can be converted to either fat or carbohydrate. That's wonderful because it means that if you don't eat any fat or carbohydrate, then a big part of the protein you consume will have to be converted to these other food elements. In the process, a lot of energy will be lost forever since the conversion process burns up a large amount of calories in the various chemical reactions. That means that simply eating only protein will give you the weight reduction benefits of exercise without lifting a finger. (Don't use this as an excuse for not exercising but you can benefit from it nevertheless.) You can literally burn up calories just by sitting down at the table and eating!

3. Since the breakdown of protein to form fat and carbohydrate is a recognized and accepted scientific fact, you can utilize a high protein intake to increase the metabolization of these food elements. The old saying, "Carbohydrate and fat burn in the flame of protein," takes on a completely new meaning.

4. In addition, protein has excellent satiety value. If you eat a slice or two of bread, in a few minutes you are hungry again. But if you eat a plate of fish or half a chicken or a piece of steak, you feel full and satisfied. In a real sense, protein "sticks to your ribs". So all we have to do is find an appetiz-ing and palatable high protein diet and we are on our way. If we follow it carefully, our weight loss will be painless and guaranteed. It just so happens that I've prepared exactly that diet for us. Let's go on to the next paragraph and see how easy it is:

DAVID REUBEN, M.D.

Basically **Module Four** or the "Super-Protein" diet, consists of high-quality protein foods arranged in appetizing forms. Here is a list of the basic components:

1. *Chicken or Turkey* ... We will only use these birds—instead of goose or duck—because they have the smallest amount of relative body fat. To eliminate even the small amount of fat chicken and turkey have, it is best to remove the skin and the fat that lies just under it before you cook them. (Some people even use a razor blade to remove every last bit of fat.) You can prepare them any way you want provided you don't use any oil, fat, or grease in the process.
2. *Meat* ... We can use any kind of meat in this Module except pork but all the fat has to be removed before cooking. You must be very careful with ground meat unless you grind it yourself since you've probably noticed that most store-ground meat contains generous amounts of fat. Again, you can cook it any way you like provided you don't use any oil, fat, or grease while you are doing it.
3. *Sea Food* ... You can eat anything in this category including lobsters, oysters, clams, squid, shrimps, crabs, and all the rest. Just be sure not to add any type of fat to them anywhere along the line.
4. *Fish* ... This is where you can really live it up. Choose any of the vast variety of fish and enjoy it—but just don't let a drop of fat touch it before it touches your lips.
5. *Cheese* ... Cheese is one of our best friends in this Module provided we only eat *skimmed milk* cheeses. That means cheese that is made entirely from skimmed milk. ("Partly skimmed milk cheese" just won't do the trick.) That means you can eat lots of nice cheeses like cottage cheese, farmer cheese, pot cheese and any hard or semi-soft cheese—just so long as they are made only with skimmed milk.

I think that's pretty good news right there—but what comes next is even better. You can eat as much as any of these food items as you want! Just like **Module One**, **Module Four** allows you an unlimited intake of any of the foods in the module. There's only one little thing that you have to be sure to do: drink plenty of water. You will need to drink at least 10 glasses of water every twenty-four hours to get the full benefit of this module. You won't find it difficult at all once you get into the habit and when you see all that weight coming off, you'll be eager to help yourself wash away all that fat, as it were.

Wash away fat? Well, that's not exactly the physiological mechanism that's at work but in the figurative sense, that's just the way it is. Since you are burning your fat away in the incandescent flame of protein metabolism, the water you drink washes away the metabolic products that you don't need or want.

I can see the next question forming on your lips: "What's the difference between this Module and **Module One**?" Here's the answer. **Module Four** is a faster and more efficient Module for more advanced dieters. You can expect more dramatic results for several reasons.

First, you know what *The Diet of Diets* program is all about and you don't need the psychological reassurance of moderate fat intake to prevent the anxiety that comes with the first Module of a dramatic new diet concept.

Secondly, **Module Four** has a much lower proportion of fat than **Module One**. Is that a surprise? Well, animal tissue—that is, meat—contains a certain amount of fat deposited in among the muscle fibers. In a piece of beef with no discernible fat whatsoever, the fat content is about 12%, so there is fat in every cut of meat, even if you can't see it with the naked eye. In chicken the percentage is somewhat less—about 8%—and in fish—codfish, for example—there is about 5% invisible fat.

There is another nice advantage to **Module Four**. It is closer to the real world. Once we return to our normal weight, we are going to eat normally and still maintain our new slim weight—that's the secret of Module Eight. Obviously we aren't going to be able to do that on a moderate fat diet so **Module Four** is a wonderful transitional diet that is going to help us advance psychologically at the same time we slim down metabolically.

Now, how about some sample menus? By now we're experts in diets and just by skimming over the outline of a diet we can get a pretty good idea of what to expect. In **Module Four**, you can pretty well set up your own menu plans without any difficulty. But just for fun, here are some examples to get you started.

BREAKFAST

A nice two-egg omelet—made in one of those wonderful non-stick frying pans. (You can have two omelets if you feel like it ...)
(Sprinkle a little fresh parsley over it if you prefer.)
A good helping of cottage cheese—as much as you like
Coffee or tea—without milk or sugar—as much as you like

LUNCH

Prime rib with fresh horseradish—as much as you like
A few good slices of a nice skimmed-milk cheddar cheese
Coffee or tea—without milk or sugar

SUPPER

Baked cod with lemon juice—as much as you like
Cottage cheese sprinkled with dried mixed herbs Italian style
Coffee or tea—without milk or sugar

In between meals you can eat as often and as much as you like, so long as you eat items in this module. A snack of cold chicken, a plate of pot cheese with dried fennel sprinkled over the top—whatever you fancy. You can also have as much tea or coffee as you wish, without cream or sugar, of course.

Here's another sample menu:

BREAKFAST

Broiled fresh salmon—as much as you like
Two "fried" eggs made in the non-stick pan
Farmer cheese. Coffee or tea—without milk or sugar

LUNCH

Cold shrimp plate with lemon juice and spices
Hard boiled eggs sliced and placed around the edges of the plate
Coffee or tea—without milk or sugar

SUPPER

> Broiled chicken with herb sauce—as much as you like
> Any solid skimmed milk cheese
> Coffee or tea—without milk or sugar

As usual, as many daytime or bedtime or midnight snacks as you wish, so long as they are from items in the Module.

I know. This is the least diversified of all the modules. *But it is the module that pays the most dividends.* In the space of a single week—a mere 21 meals—some people have been able to lose eight or even ten pounds! And remember, that's eight to ten pounds without being hungry, without taking any drugs, and without a single second of hunger. That's a week of constant eating—if that's what you want to do—and of constant weight loss.

But there's even better news. Because of the modular structure of *The Diet of Diets*, if there's any Module that doesn't appeal to you for any reason, you can just skip it and substitute another Module that you really like. So if **Module Four** seems a bit strenuous for you, you can select another Module to take its place. But before you do that, at least give it a try. I'm sure that after a day or two you will be so delighted with the results that you will want to make **Module Four** an integral part of *The Diet of Diets*.

Now the final question: Is **Module Four** safe? The answer is an unqualified "yes". As a matter of fact, **Module Four** is so safe that it's a standard diet in many Medical Centers around the world for patients who have been badly burned or who have had severe tissue injuries in aircraft or automobile accidents. In medical terminology, it is an "anabolic" diet—designed to encourage tissue repair and rapidly improve the patients strength and resistance to disease. With that in mind, you will probably notice what other *The Diet of Diets* friends have noticed. Within a few days of starting **Module Four**, they were amazed at the sudden increase in their physical strength and endurance. (Incidentally, that's the reason **Module Four** is the favorite diet of champion Olympic weight-lifters and wrestlers.) You will also find that your resistance to colds and minor illnesses will increase dramatically during the time you are on **Module Four**!

So, give it a try and you'll be delighted. Now on to our next exciting step in *The Diet of Diets*, **Module Five**!

7

Meet The Men Who Made You Fat:

"The Pixel Boys"

If you have ever had a problem with your weight, if you have ever struggled desperately and unsuccessfully to shed unwanted pounds, if you have wanted to be thin but couldn't be thin—if you have ever wished that there were someone you could blame, I have the answer to your prayers. There is group of people in this world—whose name you have never heard—who might be the object of your wrath. Everyone who drags his flab to bed at night and then again to the breakfast table in the morning may well hold a grudge against this gentleman. Everyone who eats when he doesn't feel hungry has felt the shadow of the imperceptible brilliance of a man they never met. The name of that unknown genius is none other than: **The Pixel Boys**.

You say you've never heard of them? Perhaps not, but at this very moment in your own home—not too far from your kitchen—sits the infernal device that they planted there. Their brilliant invention operates automatically and relentlessly to allow people to make you eat things you don't want to eat when you're not even hungry. Their ingenious combination of sophisticated technology and brilliant inspiration helps others to make you fatter with each hour of exposure to it. If someone could only think of a machine to fatten hogs the way their machine fattens human beings, they could name their own price—and it would be in the billions. What did **The Pixel Boys** invent? They invented the television set. They are the father of modern electronic television—in living color and stereo sound.

Of course, it didn't really happen that way. **The Pixel Boys** was actually a large group of distinguished scientists who struggled hard and long to perfect the miracle of modern television.

Obviously they had no intention to make anyone fat or unhappy. Their extraordinary invention was designed to make the world a better place for all of us. But the simple fact is that advertisements for food products on television have more impact than in any other medium and can literally make you eat things you don't want to eat when you're not even hungry. Think about it a moment or two and you'll see what I mean:

It's eight-fifteen in the evening. At six-forty P.M. you had a nice big meal—roast beef, baked potatoes, peas and carrots, two pieces of bread, and a nice big slice of chocolate cake for dessert.

Calorie-wise you have stocked up for at least three days. You're enjoying an exciting movie when there is a pause for a commercial. It's a beautiful young girl in swim suit at the edge of a pool and it has something to do with cookies and a handsome young man. There is soft music in the background with a steady slow monotonous beat and a slight flicker in the picture—that doesn't come from your set.

The camera pans first to her face, then to his face, then to her breasts and then to his swim trunks. Slowly he munches the cookie and the commercial fades away.

Suddenly you want a cookie. You don't know why and you don't care. All you know is that *you want a cookie!* You *really* want a cookie. While you may not be prepared to kill for it, you are very interested in a cookie. If there is a cookie within reach you will eat it. If not, you will probably eat the closest thing you can find to a cookie whether it is another slice of chocolate cake, a piece of candy, or a dish of ice cream. But your cookie-appetite has been touched off and you must heed the call.

An exaggeration? Hardly. It happens to all of us—and not just with cookies, It happens with soft drinks, with beer, with wine, with potato chips, with pizza, with bread, with meat, with anything that can be eaten and sold via television. And that means everything. How does it happen? Very simple. You are invited to participate in an electronic hallucination.

That's right, an hallucination. That's what television is. You experience—with your senses—something that isn't happening. You see a girl and a boy, you hear them talking, you see them eating, you hear music—and none of it really exists.

What you are reacting to is a flicker of thousands of little lights going on and off on the surface of a glowing phosphorescent electronic tube in a darkened room. The girl isn't there, the boy isn't there and the cookie isn't there. It's all just a bunch of electrical charges dancing around in a big glass bulb. But the hallucination is designed and constructed with such genius that you experience it as if it were actually happening. Then something else happens. You fall into a hypnotic trance.

Does that sound crazy? Well, it's not. Oh, I know, you don't slide off your favorite chair onto the floor. You don't turn into a robot lurching into the kitchen to obediently eat everything on the third shelf of the refrigerator. You don't start mumbling things like, "I await your instructions, Master ..." Maybe they could do it if they wanted to but that's not what the cookie people are aiming for.

They just want to inflame your appetite for cookies—preferably their brand of cookies. In hypnosis, there are many levels of hypnotic trance, from the lightest to the most profound. As you read these pages, if you really get into them, you enter a superficial level of hypnosis that we call "concentration". You shut out most external stimuli and focus all your attention on what you are reading. When people watch television, they do the same thing, only more so. If you don't believe me, just sneak a glance at your friends when they are watching their favorite programs. Their eyes are wide, their stares are fixed, their mouths droop open, and they react emotionally to what they see. Occasionally they will smile or wince or frown—depending on what the electrons are doing on the surface of the little glass bulb. That is hypnosis.

There are a lot of things that one can do to increase or decrease the level of hypnosis produced by electronic hallucinations such as television. If the action is jerky and uncoordinated, if the sounds are annoying and discordant, if the images are bright and intrusive, the level of hypnosis is very slight. But if the images are soft and shadowy, if the music is monotonous and rhythmic, if the camera moves from one "hot" area to another—lips, breasts, eyes, groin, buttocks, etc.— then the level of hypnosis deepens significantly. With that in mind, let's go back and take another look at the cookie commercial:

(It's eight-fifteen on a cold January evening. You have been watching an adventure movie and you are a little bit excited. Now suddenly the movie cuts off and the commercial fills the screen.)

A lovely blonde girl in a mini-bikini is lying on her back with her eyes closed at the side of a swimming pool. There are palm trees in the background and all the trappings of a luxurious tropical estate. The camera slowly moves from her feet up to her head, stopping briefly at her pubic area and her breasts. In the background, very soft percussion music with a tropical beat is playing:

Da-da-dum … Da-da-dum … Da-da-dum …

Suddenly there is a fast jump-cut to the other side of the pool. A man's legs, from the calves down, are walking toward the girl. They move in time to the music in a kind of sensual prance—like a tiger's paws. The camera follows the legs for a few moments and then suddenly cuts to a darkly handsome man kneeling over the supine beauty. He looks her over from down to up as the camera follows his gaze: legs, pubis, breasts, lips. The camera slides over his body gently, lingering a moment at his crotch. The whole thing is done so subtly that you are hardly aware of it—consciously.

Then he leans over to kiss her on the lips—her eyes are still closed. He closes his eyes and just as their lips are about to make contact, she suddenly reaches up and pops a cookie into his mouth! She raises her head, smiles mischievously into the camera and winks. He chews the cookie contentedly and looks upward, rolling his eyes in pleasure. With a final loud *Da-da-dum*! of the music, you are released from your hypnotic experience and handed back to the adventure movie. Want a cookie now?

What happened to you? Nothing much. You were just hypnotized. The steady beat of the music, the flicker in the picture, and the slow lazy camera movement lulled you into a moderate hypnotic trance. Then you were eased into a tropical love fantasy with powerful sexual stimulation—breasts, crotch, lips—and at the last moment a cookie was substituted for the impending sexual satisfaction.

The message was carefully shaped—if you can't have an orgasm, at least you can have a cookie. Before you could protest, you were awakened with a loud *Da-da-dum*! of the hypnotic music and delivered back to reality. Of course you wanted a cookie. You *had* to want a cookie.

This message is repeated at least 200 times a day for the average city dweller—in big metropolitan areas it can hit you as much as 1000 times in twenty-four hours. Let's just go through an ordinary day. When your clock radio wakes you up, the first thing you hear in the morning is a commercial for breakfast cereal and an artificial orange drink. Then to the breakfast table and the morning paper.

You will probably see some ads for bread and muffins, marmalade, and bacon. (The food advertisers know that some people read the paper at breakfast.) If you watch TV at breakfast, you will see plenty of breakfast cereal ads, imitation orange drink ads, and pork sausage ads. (The food advertisers know that some people watch TV at breakfast.) Then it's off to work. As you drive through the crowded streets listening to the car radio, you hear one commercial after another for food and drink.

Most of them have a sexual undertone—soft female voices, sexy music, invitations to sexually-tinged adventures. From the car you can see billboards advertising food and drink as well—usually with more or less undressed females to get your attention. By the time you arrive at work you can hardly wait for the coffee break—and you don't know why. Or at least you didn't know why until now.

That barrage of intense brainwashing goes on throughout your day—and most of the time you're not even aware that it's happening. If you want to have a little fun, one day just add up all the exposures you have to food advertising and you'll be surprised. Be sure to count every impact that a food ad makes on you—from store window displays to posters to billboards to magazines to radio to television and all the rest. I think you will be truly amazed.

Now what does this all mean for us dieters? It means trouble, that's what it means. No matter how much we may be dedicated to our diets, no matter how powerful our devotion to losing weight, we are being constantly deluged by super-sophisticated psychological motivation compelling us to eat when we don't want to eat, when we don't need to eat, and when we shouldn't eat.

What are we going to do about it? We are going to defend ourselves against it, that's what we are going to do about it.

We are going to develop a freedom-fighter mentality to struggle against the powerful forces that threaten our health and slimness. Every time we see a food ad—wherever it occurs—we are going to steel ourselves against its effect. The most powerful and dangerous ads—to a dieter—are those on television because of their intensity and subtlety. At the beginning of a diet, it is really best not to watch too much TV. That's the moment when we are most vulnerable and when we have the most to lose. The same is true of magazines that are replete with irresistible food ads. Just let them go until we have our weight under control. This is the moment when it is better to read books and listen to music than to devote ourselves entirely to magazines and television. It is also a good idea not to read about food when we are eating. That's the ideal situation for a food advertiser—get to the consumer when he is consuming. So, the key to success in defending ourselves against the hypnosis of food advertising is awareness and avoidance. And the key to success in slimming down awaits us in **Module Five**—which follows immediately.

Module Five is one of my favorites. It is refreshing, invigorating, and full of energy. It makes you feel good at the same time it peels off the pounds. It also makes you noticeably healthier and younger-looking. You can see the results in the glow of health in your skin, in the spring in your step, and in the renewed capacity for work and fun that you will experience.

As with most Modules on *The Diet of Diets*, **Module Five** allows you to eat as much as you want anytime—with no limit and no restriction. I know you're going to enjoy it and the only problem you might have is giving it up when your twenty-one meals are over. It's possible to extend it of course, if you feel that strongly about it. By now I'm sure you're wondering why we call it, "Always Springtime …"

Well, here's the answer. The entire content of **Module Five** is Springtime. It is fresh and light and fragrant. It never makes you feel heavy or drugged. It satisfies you and lightens you and purifies you—all at the same time. And after a long hard winter of overweight, it brings the promise of a warm and gentle summer of health and slimness. Here it is:

On **Module Five** you can eat as much as you want of any kind of fruit or vegetable—without any limit whatsoever. You can use any spices you desire in any amount. You can drink tea or coffee—without milk or sugar—or mineral water without limit.

When you make salads, you should use only fresh lemon juice or the best quality vinegar as a dressing. Don't use any dried fruits or vegetables—*fresh* is the key word always on **Module Five**. You can fry certain vegetables according to the recipes in the chapter on recipes but always use a non-stick frying pan and no grease or oil. Here are a few basic rules to follow but beyond that, your imagination can run free— and you can have the gastronomic adventure of your life! Here are the simple rules:

1. Everything on your diet should be *fresh*. There is no place for canned, dried bottled, frozen, or otherwise embalmed food on this diet. There is a good reason for that. Fresh food is far more nutritious and filling than processed food and keeps you safe from potentially harmful food additives. It may seem to be more expensive to buy fresh fruits and vegetables but it is much cheaper than buying medicine, paying doctors, and staying in the hospital. After all, weight reduction is really therapy for your health and your happiness—the best investment you can ever make.

2. Everything you choose should be absolutely the best quality available. Pick the best and ripest apples and pears. Choose the nicest mushrooms and celery. Treat yourself to the most luscious tomatoes and lettuce. You deserve it and it will go a long way to make **Module Five** successful and enjoyable.

3. If you can, eat everything raw and unpeeled. In many cases the most important nutrients in fruits and vegetables are in the part that we are used to throwing away. It's what we throw in the garbage that has the nutrition and what we serve on our tables that sometimes we should be throwing away. An excellent example is the skin of the potato. The potato skin— which usually ends up in the garbage can—contains the following essential nutrients:

   1. Ten per cent of the **protein** of the potato.

2. Twenty per cent of the **fiber** of the potato.

3. Sixteen per cent of the **calcium** of the potato.

4. Twenty-six per cent of the **phosphorus** of the potato.

5. Sixteen per cent of the **iron** of the potato.

6. Thirty per cent of the **potassium** of the potato.

7. Twenty-five per cent of **riboflavin** of the potato.

8. Twenty-per cent of the **niacin** of the potato.

If we throw the potato skin away, that's how much we lose!

Almost all other fruits and vegetables tell us the same story. Of course you don't want to eat orange peels or pineapple skins, for obvious reasons. But whenever you can, eat the peel!

The same logic applies to eating fruits and vegetables raw. No matter how you do it and no matter what anyone tells you, cooking destroys nutrients in food. Take the humble garden pea. A raw pea is a thing of delight and a joy forever. With its unsurpassable tart-sweet flavor and its rich non-fattening natural sweetness, it is unequaled in the world of garden vegetables. Now boil that pea and see what happens:

It loses, in the process of being boiled alive, the following vital nutrients:

1. Fifteen per cent of all its **protein**.

2. Thirteen per cent of all its **carbohydrate**.

3. Eleven per cent of all its **calcium**.

4. Fifteen per cent of all its **phosphorus**.

5. Five per cent of all its **iron**.

6. A whopping thirty-seven per cent of all its **potassium**!

7. Sixteen per cent of all its **vitamin A**.

8. Twenty per cent of all its **vitamin B1 (thiamine)**.

9. Twenty-one per cent of all its **riboflavin**.

10. Twenty per cent of all its **niacin**.

11. And finally, twenty-six per cent of all its **vitamin C**!

Was it worth it? Hardly.

The noble pea also offers us an opportunity to observe the massive destruction that occurs when a fresh vegetable is canned. Compared to a fresh pea, a canned pea has lost forever, the following vital nutrients:

1. Twenty-five per cent of all its **protein**.
2. Thirty-one per cent of all its **phosphorus**.
3. A terrifying seventy per cent loss of all its vital **potassium**!
4. A shocking seventy-four per cent loss of all its **vitamin B**
5. A fifty-seven per cent loss of all its **riboflavin**!
6. A massive seventy-two per cent loss of all its **niacin**!
7. An astounding seventy per cent loss of all its **vitamin C**!

To be absolutely complete, there is one thing that a canned pea offers you that no fresh pea ever could:

A massive dose of salt! The sodium content of the average canned pea is a mere *two hundred and thirty-nine thousand per cent higher* than a fresh pea. For anyone with a tendency toward heart disease or water retention, that can mean the difference between happiness and misery. Knowing that, why should anyone in the world ever want to eat a canned pea?

    4. Eat until you are full and then stop eating. That makes all the sense in the world, doesn't it? And with **Module Five** you never have to stock up for the future since you always know that you can go back and eat more anytime you want it—morning, noon, or night or even at three in the morning.

There are some other sensational advantages to **Module Five**. Your problems of water retention could be solved once and for all. The combination of vitamins and minerals and enzymes in **Module Five** provide a natural stimulus to the loss of retained fluids that is unequaled anywhere. You will not only be trim and slim, you should be absolutely un-waterlogged! One of the most annoying problems of traditional weight reduction programs, constipation, is eliminated from the very first day on **Module Five**. Because of its high fiber content, constipation is literally impossible on this very excellent Module.

Now let's get to the fun part—let's have a look at some sample menus:

BREAKFAST

Sliced oranges with freshly-grated coconut sprinkled on top
Juicy purple plums

Watermelon rounds
Tea or coffee in any amount—without milk or sugar

LUNCH

Springtime Salad: Lettuce, asparagus spears, tomatoes, shredded carrots with fresh lemon juice dressing and crushed thyme and rosemary sprinkled on top.
A bowlful of immense luscious ripe peaches
Tea or coffee in any amount—without milk or sugar

SUPPER

Perfectly ripe melon with fresh lemon juice
Eggplant and tomato casserole with Oriental spices (see recipe chapter ...)
Crispy baked potato skins
Tea or coffee in any amount—without milk or sugar

LATE NIGHT SNACK

Crisp tart apples

If you still worry about calories in weight reduction, you will enjoy seeing the calorie count for these three ample meals plus the late night snack. The *total calorie count* is—hang on to your hat—*six hundred and forty* tiny *calories for the entire day!*

That's for an awful lot of food. Even if you could somehow force yourself to eat six meals and two snacks a day on **Module Five**, you would still only be consuming 1280 calories for the day. But no one in their right mind can eat that much food—and that's your immense margin of safety on **Module Five**. You just can't overeat the massive physical volume and bulk of this delightful Module.

Let's look at another day's sample menu:

BREAKFAST

Ripe pink grapefruit
Pink Papaya with fresh lemon juice
Tea or coffee in any amount—without milk or sugar

LUNCH

Coleslaw with cider vinegar and fresh grapes and celery seeds (see recipe chapter …)
Corn-on-the-cob
Fresh sliced giant tomatoes
Tea or coffee in any amount—without milk or sugar

SUPPER

Sautéed fresh mushrooms with freshly-ground pepper and natural spices (use a non-stick frying pan and no grease …)
Beets and watercress marinade (see recipe chapter …)
Tea or coffee in any amount—without milk or sugar

LATE NIGHT SNACK

Fresh pineapple slices

For today the grand total is *four hundred and fifty-five* tiny *calories*! If you went crazy and somehow ate six meals and three snacks on this excellent Module, you still couldn't go over 1365 total calories that day. But you will find that the three meals and a snack are more than enough to satisfy you both nutritionally and emotionally.

Here are a few hints that will make **Module Five** even more exciting and appetizing. Use your food blender and food processor constantly and creatively. You can make fruit drinks and combinations limited only by your imagination. Salads can be your greatest satisfaction since you have the entire world of fruits and vegetables to work with. Don't be afraid to try new fruits and new vegetables— including ones that you don't even know the names of. Ask your grocer and your friends and you will be amazed at the new and exciting discoveries you will make. Now let's ask and answer the question that always comes up with **Module Five**:

"Since this is a vegetarian diet, isn't there some risk of vitamin or protein deficiency?"

The answer is a resounding "NO!" Here are the reasons for it:

1. This diet, **Module Five**, is so packed with vitamins and minerals that you will be getting ten times as much of these

elements as your neighbor who is on a standard meat-and-potatoes diet. He's the one who is running the risks, not you.

2. Fruits and vegetables contain large amounts of protein. You will be eating complementary combinations of many different fruits and vegetables and your protein intake should be quite satisfactory.

3. Remember that more than half the population of this planet lives very nicely on virtually nothing but fruits and vegetables—and they are slimmer and healthier than most of us.

4. Many of the Olympic Gold Medal endurance event winners are vegetarians. No one can fault them when it comes to strength, health, and endurance. They must know something about diet that the average person hasn't discovered yet.

5. As always, in *The Diet of Diets*, you only follow each Module for a mere 21 meals. You could go without eating anything for 21 meals and suffer no ill effects whatsoever. But in this case you are eating vast amounts of the highest quality food known to the human race. There is nothing to worry about.

So be calm and confident as you set out on **Module Five**, "Always Springtime …", and within the first few days into the Module, that's the way you'll be feeling!

8

Get Milk? But Why?

Milk, milk, milk! Sometimes it seems that this whole world of ours revolves around milk! We are constantly deluged with propaganda from all sides telling us to drink milk.

"Fresh milk makes healthy babies!" "Milk is your best food!" "Drink your quart of milk today!" We have powdered milk, skimmed milk, powdered skimmed milk, buttermilk, acidophilus milk, evaporated milk, condensed milk, raw milk, homogenized milk, pasteurized milk, ultra-high temperature milk, chocolate milk, milk chocolate, milk shakes, malted milk, ice milk, ice cream, cream, whipped cream, sour cream, and every other possible combination of milk and milk products you can imagine.

You would think that our moment-to-moment survival depended on a constant infusion of milk. It almost seems as if milk is as important to us as the air we breathe. Well, in a way, it is.

From the first drink of mother's milk or formula milk when we enter this existence to the last sip of warm sugared milk as we leave for a better world, milk occupies center stage in the on-going drama of human nutrition. It is as if we had built a special religion around that thin white fluid. The first few years of our lives revolve around milk. In the beginning we hardly drink or eat anything else. It's milk six times a day and that's about it. Later we start in on milk puddings, creamy dishes, butter on our bread, and the ever present glass of milk at every meal. Almost all our associations with milk are pleasant ones—security, contentment, being with Mother, and to top it all off, a nice clean taste.

That's the reason why milk, above and beyond all the rest of its qualities, has the ability to *satisfy*. When you are tired, when you are tense, when you are worried, a nice glass of milk can do wonders to calm you down. When you can't sleep, a nice warm glass of milk can put you to sleep like a baby. Hold on! What did we just say? "Can put you to sleep like a baby?" But isn't that what used to happen?

Whenever Mommy wanted to put you to sleep, all she had to do was pop a nursing bottle of nice warm milk into your little baby mouth and you nodded off in two shakes of a lamb's tail.

Remember a few years back how all the great geniuses were predicting that "modern science" would soon make discoveries that would allow us to stop eating. All we were going to do was pop one little pill three times a day and we wouldn't have to eat any more. Then we wouldn't have to be bothered with such nuisances as roast beef, southern fried chicken, baked ham, steamed lobster, chocolate mousse and about 25,000 other delightful dishes. Fortunately something distracted that army of scientific geniuses and they never got around to perfecting those horrible little pills that were going to do away with good eating forever. Even if they had succeeded, the project would have been a colossal flop. Because we don't eat to get vitamins and minerals and calories. We eat to get satisfaction! And as I'm sure you've noticed, pills don't satisfy.

So, to be successful, a reducing diet has to fill us without fattening us, satisfy us without stuffing us, and meet all our nutritional needs at the same time. Is there such a diet? Well, you know I wouldn't have asked you that question if I didn't have a Module like that up my sleeve. But before we get to that part, let's ask ourselves another question:

A lot of people have written a lot of things about milk and a lot of things about food but probably the most fascinating assertion of all is the one that states that "Milk is the perfect food!" If that's true, it's bound to be the most interesting fact in the entire history of human nutrition. Let's take a look at it:

Nutritional Values of "fresh" milk ...

(per 100 grams or 3½ ounces)

water: 85%
sodium: 16 mg
calories: 77
potassium: 51 mg
protein: 1.1 g
vitamin A: 240 IU
fat: 4%
thiamine (vitamin B1): 0.01 mg
carbohydrate: 9.5%
riboflavin: 0.04 mg
calcium: 33 mg
niacin: 0.2 mg
iron: 0.1 mg
vitamin C: 5 mg
phosphorus: 14 mg

It doesn't look too bad does it? Or does it? If we compare the nutritional value of milk with what the nutritional "experts" say we should be eating, we might be in for a little trouble.

Brace yourself for the bad news. According to the rigid nutritional standards, established by the so-called "experts" in nutrition, milk is a total flop! It has too little water, too many calories, too little protein, too much fat, much too much carbohydrate, inadequate potassium, not nearly enough calcium, and insufficient riboflavin and niacin. To make matters worse, it isn't homogenized or pasteurized! To tell the truth, in most modern countries of the world, you wouldn't even be allowed to sell it!

But I'm not talking about just any old milk. The chart you see above shows the nutritional value of human milk—the most perfect combination of nutritional elements ever provided for the human race. Far better than any concoction that comes from the mind of man, human milk is the only nutrient that can honestly be described as "the perfect food".

Because our original experience with Mother's milk—or its subsequent substitutes—was so satisfying emotionally, we have spent our lives seeking the same satisfaction from other less natural derivatives of the watery white fluid. It's amazing, if you stop to think about it, how much of our milk consumption is "recreational" and not nutritional. For example, the very sweet "milk chocolate", which contains small amounts of actual milk, is the largest selling type of chocolate in the world. Vanilla ice cream outsells all other flavors by far and is the closest counterfeit in terms of appearance and flavor to Mother's milk.

Over-sweetened whipped cream appears almost everywhere as a luxury item. Cloyingly sweet chocolate-flavored milk is a favorite drink of small children who still yearn nostalgically for Mother's breast milk. Almost all the milk by-products that we eat in quantity tend to duplicate the sweetness and smoothness of Mother's milk. Almost everyone who has a weight problem consumes excessive amounts of imitations of Mother's milk, in one form or another, smuggled in as "food for grown- ups".

There is no question that one of the biggest problems that confronts serious dieters like us is the temptation to over-consume sweets. We can eat a big meal, adhering strictly to whatever weight-loss diet we may be following and for some terrible reason, we just don't feel satisfied! But as soon as we swallow a few bites (or maybe more …) of milk chocolate, we suddenly feel satisfied and contented.

We can be on our diets for a week or so, never deviating by even so much as a mouthful, when suddenly the craving for a dish of ice cream attacks us. That's it! One tiny spoonful turns into a dozen not-so-tiny spoonfuls and before we know it, the pint of ice cream is almost gone. How do we feel? You know that I hate to say it and I know that you hate to hear me say it. But I have to tell the truth. *We feel great! We feel wonderful! We feel super!*

Why? Because we have just had our "milk fix". For the same reason that babies go right to sleep after nursing, we are calmed and tranquillized by our desperately-needed dose of milk. The next morning, however, is a different story. As we creep onto the bathroom scale, the reproach rings in our ears: "Why did you do it?" "Look at all the weight you've put on!" To us, like to every addict, the dawn brings remorse.

What's the solution? Well, just as in every serious problem, there are many possible solutions. We can simply surrender ourselves to the milk-craving and spend the rest of our lives wallowing in syrupy-sweet milk derivatives up to our double-chins. We will put on weight like a water-buffalo but at least we will have milk constantly on our lips—for the few years that we are likely to survive, that is. Or we can grit our teeth and clench our fists and renounce, once and for all, milk in any form.

We may become melancholy and disagreeable to everyone around us, we may go for long solitary walks and occasionally bay at the moon, but we can be arrogant and proud that we have not succumbed to the lure of imitation Mother's milk. Fortunately, there is a third solution. We can confront the problem of milk honestly with all its nostalgia and yearning and secret satisfaction and find a way to resolve it once and for all. Then it will never be a problem again.

We can take our greatest temptation and turn it around so that it is our greatest ally in our constant war against overweight. We can take a deep breath and descend into that shadowy valley of milk and baby and Mother once again and come out on the other side, cheerful, victorious, and confident. And incidentally, much thinner than when we went in.

How are we going to do that? We are going to plunge fearlessly into **Module Six**—one of our greatest and most rewarding adventures in the exciting *The Diet of Diets*!

What we are going to find in **Module Six** is really the answer to every dieter's prayers. We are going to find a diet that is eminently satisfying—both to mind and body—and that fills every possible nutritional need at the same time. In addition—and at no extra charge, as they say on television, **Module Six** is going to peel off the pounds beyond our wildest dreams. There are also some other superb and unexpected fringe benefits. For those of us who have trouble falling asleep at night, **Module Six** is going to put us into the Land of Nod as quick as our heads hit the pillow. Why? Listen to this for a fascinating sidelight.

Module Six has as yet-to-be-discovered secret ingredient, perhaps an enzyme that overwhelms insomnia like nothing else known. So if you ever have the slightest trouble getting to sleep, plug into **Module Six** and your troubles will be over. There's something else that is very special about **Module Six**. It produces what we doctors call "euphoria". (You know that doctors can't call things by the same names as regular people do. That would make medicine sound too easy.)

Euphoria is simply feeling wonderful. When someone is euphoric, nothing bothers them. The car payment can be overdue, the dog may have chewed up your best Italian shoes, the FBI is ringing your doorbell—and you couldn't care less. As far as you're concerned things are wonderful and getting better. That's only a sample of what you can expect on **Module Six**.

Okay, now how do we do all that? Well, one way might be to get you back on Mother's milk again. Theoretically, that should solve all your problems but there are some practical considerations. First and foremost, your consumption has jumped quite a bit since you first weighed in at six pounds four ounces. Where do you get your daily supply of three liters of Mother's milk? Secondly, there is a significant shortage of women who are willing to supply the product.

Babies usually come in serial form, one after the other, so that Mothers rarely have to contend with the problem of feeding three at once, much less thirteen at a time. So we can discard forever the thought of going back to the original—and undoubtedly most satisfying—arrangement of Mother's milk. What we really need to do is find some other form of milk that will be nearly as good. Let's take a look at plain old cow's milk. Here's the way it checks out:

Nutritional Values of cow's milk ...

(per 100 grams or 3½ ounces)

> water: 87%
> sodium: 50 mg
> calories: 65
> potassium: 144 mg
> protein: 3.5 g
> vitamin A: 140 IU
> fat: 3.5%
> thiamine (vitamin B1): 0.03 mg
> carbohydrate: 4.9%

riboflavin: 0.17 mg
calcium: 118 mg
niacin: 0.1 mg
iron: trace
vitamin C: 1 mg
phosphorus: 93 mg

That's not too bad but to tell you the truth, I'm not exactly overwhelmed with the benefits of ordinary cow's milk for adult human beings. For one thing, it really has too many calories. I know we don't waste a lot of time worrying about an extra calorie here or an extra calorie there, but sixty-five big calories in a mere 100 grams is pushing it a bit too hard. I'm not, shall we say, euphoric about the fat content either.

A rapidly-growing baby can use a good dose of fat in his daily diet but three-and-a-half per cent is too much for you and me. The amount of vitamin A is totally insignificant since the daily requirement, according to the textbooks is a whopping 5000 IU.

Therefore, the difference between 240 Units of the vitamin in Mother's milk and 140 Units in cow's milk is minuscule. Likewise the difference between one milligram of Vitamin C and five milligrams of Vitamin C doesn't really amount to anything since the purported daily requirement of Vitamin C is at least 50 milligrams. But the excess of calories and the overabundance of fat makes ordinary cow's milk just not right for us on **Module Six**.

What to do? Well, there are some advantages to goat's milk and buffalo milk has several unique qualities (in all seriousness, since we never joke about such important things …) but these otherwise desirable milks just aren't available to most of us. So we have to cast about for a milk that is abundant, available, reasonably-priced and that gives us most of the qualities of Mother's milk. But we also need a milk that is up-dated for the benefit of weight-conscious adults like you and I.

Is there such a product?. If there were, it would be the answer to a dieters dream. Well, you know I wouldn't have brought you this far if I didn't have just what you need right up my sleeve. Here it is. The formula that is closest to Mother's milk and adapted to the needs of the weight-conscious adult:

Here's the formula:

Nutritional Values of "special" milk ...

(per 100 grams or 3½ ounces)

> water: 90.5%
> sodium: 130 mg
> calories: 36
> potassium: 140 mg
> protein: 3.6 g
> vitamin A: trace
> fat: 0.1%
> thiamine (vitamin B1): 0.04 mg
> carbohydrate: 5.1%
> riboflavin: 0.18 mg
> calcium: 121 mg
> niacin: 0.1 mg
> iron: trace
> vitamin C: 1 mg
> phosphorus: 95 mg

As you let your eyes dance over these wonderful figures I am sure you are as excited as I am! Look how perfect it is for what we want to accomplish! Over ninety per cent water! Three and a half ounces only contain a mere 36 calories! The fat content is an infinitesimal one-tenth of one per cent! There is four times the calcium of Mother's milk as well as four times the Vitamin B1. There is also four times the riboflavin that Mother used to provide. It even has about six times more phosphorus than in Mother's milk.

That's excellent because it coincides with the desired ratio of calcium to phosphorus that adults require. Don't worry about the Vitamin A and the iron. It's true that there's not very much in this wonderful milk formula but we'll solve that problem in the next paragraph or so—just as we solve all such problems that might stand in the way of rapid, safe, and painless weight loss in *The Diet of Diets*.

This super milk formula also gives us about five per cent carbohydrate for a feeling of satisfaction but far less than the nine-and-a-half per cent that one gets in Mother's milk. This is really the best news any dieter could ever hope for—a superbly nutritious diet that really makes you feel good. But now to the big question—where do you find this magic concoction?

The answer? Almost anywhere. Just ask for it by its name: buttermilk. That's right. By some wonderful twist of fate, buttermilk is the one readily available formula closest to an adult version of Mother's milk. And don't think that we are going to let a magnificent coincidence like that slip through our fingers! Here's the way we're going to put it together. This is **Module Six**:

You can drink in the course of a day, six glasses of buttermilk. Be sure and drink it as cold as you can comfortably manage and space the glasses throughout the day—every two hours should be about right.

In addition you can eat as much cottage cheese as you wish. Now as with all the unlimited foods on *The Diet of Diets*, you, of course, are going to use common sense. No one who wants to lose weight will try to see how much cottage cheese they can force down their throat in twenty-four hour period just to prove that they *can* gain weight on a reducing diet. If you're willing to be very serious about it, you can even eat creamed cottage cheese.

Creamed cottage cheese has a few more calories but it is also more satisfying than the rather dry and pebbly un-creamed variety. Just for fun, here is the nutritional breakdown on the cottage cheese so that you can see how impressive the nourishment is with this particular Module:

Nutritional Values of cottage cheese ...

(per 100 grams or 3½ ounces)

water: 78.3%
sodium: 229 mg
calories: 106
potassium: 85 mg
protein: 13.6 g
vitamin A: trace
fat: 4.2%
thiamine (vitamin B1): 0.03 mg
carbohydrate: 2.9%

riboflavin: 0.25 mg

calcium: 94 mg

niacin: 0.1 mg

iron: 0.3 mg

vitamin C: 0

phosphorus: 152 mg

Look at that protein! As you know, protein is excellent for staying power. When you eat a food that is high in protein, you don't want any more to eat until the next meal. Yet, in **Module Six** you will never get too much protein. The carbohydrate is at a moderate level and the fat is well under control. You will also notice that the iron we were talking about is there.

This is one of the keys to success of **Module Six**—whatever you don't find in the buttermilk portion of this Module, you are likely to find in the cottage cheese portion. The same holds true for the Vitamin A we mentioned a couple of paragraphs back. There is 170 milligrams of Vitamin A in every 100 gram portion—fine for the week that you are going to follow **Module Six**.

There is only one other point to remember—an important detail that has become familiar to us as we have been working our way pleasantly through our *The Diet of Diets*. We have to always drink plenty of water. There is nothing like H_2O to make a diet work like it should. Every enzyme reaction in our bodies takes place in water. Every chemical reaction within our millions of body cells depends on ample amounts of water being available.

If we want to sabotage our weight loss—and our health in general—all we have to do is be careless and not provide our bodies with enough water. How much is enough? The general rule is to drink at least ten glasses a day of water—in addition to tea, coffee, soft drinks and juices. That should be enough to keep our urine absolutely water-white—the sign that our body has the water it needs for all our vital chemical reactions.

Okay, now how do we go about **Module Six**? Very easy, that's how. It's simply a matter of spacing our glasses of nice cold buttermilk throughout the day. At mealtimes we eat as much cottage cheese as we feel like and that's that. We can also have the usual coffee and tea without cream or sugar in unlimited amounts.

That's about it and that's about all we really need. This Module very quickly produces a feeling of serenity and total calm that makes food and eating seem totally unimportant. Within a day or two, you won't even care to think about what you're eating. Believe me, you're in for one of the most pleasant surprises of your life! Just for the record, here's a sample menu but you can change the times to suit your own personal schedule:

BREAKFAST

One glass of buttermilk
Creamed cottage cheese, any amount
Coffee or tea without cream or sugar

TEN A.M.

One glass of buttermilk

MID-DAY

One glass of buttermilk
Creamed cottage cheese, any amount
Coffee or tea without cream or sugar

TWO P.M.

One glass of buttermilk

SUPPER TIME

One glass of buttermilk
Creamed cottage cheese, any amount
Coffee or tea without cream or sugar

BED TIME

One glass of buttermilk

If you still like to add up the calories, **Module Six** gives some very interesting numbers. Take six big glasses of buttermilk at 85 calories each—that's 510 calories. Then take 300 grams (about ten ounces) of creamed cottage—if you can possibly put away that much in a day.

That's 318 calories more, for a total of 828 little tiny calories. And if you ever wanted to know what the word "full" meant, just try this Module.

How much can you expect to lose? Well, we both know by now that our individual weight loss depends on so many personal factors. However some people have lost as much as ten pounds in the first week on this Module while feeling full and bursting with energy. So, enjoy **Module Six** to your heart's content and as soon as you're ready for it, we'll move right on to something that's just as exciting in its own very special way—**Module Seven**!

9

The Secret Of "Insalata" That Makes You A

Winner

Has anyone ever taken the time to explore the magical appeal of salads? Even the word "salad" itself has a very special appeal—it appears in almost every language in some form. In Spanish it is "ensalada", in French, "salade", in Italian, "insalata", in German, "Salat". The original word, "salad" comes from two separate ancient languages, both of them long passed out of existence—Middle French and Old Persian. In our concept salad is based on a combination of greens plus other ingredients with a heavy dose of salt and a mixture of oil and vinegar or lemon juice.

For some reason, a salad seems to be eminently satisfying to human beings. The combination of textures, colors, and flavors, artfully intermingled, has an appeal to eaters that no other dish can possibly offer. It is as if the body was crying out for the combination of foods in the proportions that exist in salad mixtures. It is as if it needs all those vitamins and minerals and enzymes that we actually know so little about.

Are you surprised that I said, "… that we know so little about"? Well, you shouldn't be because the truth is, with all our so-called "Modern Medicine", our knowledge of nutrition is barely rudimentary.

So many of the basic concepts of "Modern Nutrition" are little more than educated guesses and it is becoming obvious that even many of those guesses are not exactly on target.

In reality no one knows what food elements a human being really requires to become healthy and to stay healthy. Virtually all of the "nutritional studies" that have been performed have been deprivation studies and almost all of them have been performed on animals. What does that mean? Well, for one thing it means that nutrition research has usually been done backwards.

Look at it this way. To find out if we need a vitamin, say, Vitamin A, researchers take a tiny mouse and deliberately give him a diet deficient in Vitamin A. Then they watch and see what happens to him. His little eyes may get red, his tiny tufts of hair may fall out, he may lose interest in eating his deficient diet. Then the researchers write down all the symptoms of the tiny rodents and then guess that the same deficiency of the same vitamin will cause the same symptoms in man. You see the problem right away.

No one deliberately eats a diet that is deficient only in Vitamin A. That's obvious. Even more obvious is the fact that mice are not people. They are mammals but then so are whales and bats and so far no one has suggested that we go on the same diet as a whale or a bat.

There's much more to it besides. In all the popular books on nutrition we read about a standard group of vitamins including the ones we have mentioned from time to time. The list includes Vitamin A, Vitamin B1, Vitamin B2, Vitamin B6, Vitamin B12, Vitamin C, Vitamin D, Vitamin E, Vitamin K, and assorted others. There is also a long list of minerals that are considered to be essential including calcium, phosphorus, iron, magnesium, potassium, and many more. We already know about the essential amino acids in detail from our study together of proteins.

Why am I telling you all this? Well, after all the time we've spent together, you can guess I am leading up to something very important. And this time it is super-important. Let's say we take an experimental animal—be it a rat, a mouse, a rabbit, a dog, or even a monkey.

Let's say we take advantage of all the latest up-to-the-minute knowledge of modern scientific nutrition. Let's say that we gather every nutrient known to modern medical science, one-by-one. Let's say that we carefully mix together all of our individual vitamins, minerals, amino acids, trace elements and all the rest to make a perfect synthetic ration.

Feed that carefully-concocted "perfect diet" to let's say, our rabbit. For a few weeks he will do very nicely. His little eyes will glow brightly, his fur will be nice and shiny, his ears will be pink and straight. But then one morning early we will pop in to see him and our little bunny will be lying there with his paws up in the air, stiff as a board, gone to Bunny Heaven. What happened? Simply this. By giving him everything that modern nutrition says is essential for his health and welfare, we have starved our bunny-rabbit to death! The absolute truth is that no one knows all the things that human beings need in their diet! Even if we feed bunnies all the things that appear in the list of "essential food elements", they will be missing a lot—and they will eventually sicken and die.

Now you can see what we have been doing without coming out and telling you. The entire structure of *The Diet of Diets* is carefully designed to help us lose weight and protect our health at the same time! The only way to make sure that a person gets all the nutrients that he needs is to insist that he eats a varied diet—a diet that includes as many different possible types of foods as possible over a period of time. Fortunately that period of time can be relatively long for almost everything we eat.

For example, if we could stop all our intake of Vitamin E today we will have to start worrying about a deficiency of Vitamin E in exactly eight years! That is, we have enough Vitamin E stored in our body fat to last us that long. Somewhat the same thing is true of Vitamins A, D, and K, also stored in our body fat. As a matter of fact, Vitamin K is manufactured inside our own large intestine! The "B" Vitamins and Vitamin C are soluble in water so we need to get them a little more frequently but to develop a true vitamin deficiency takes a lot of time and a lot of deprivation.

In *The Diet of Diets* there is never any possibility of any nutritional deficiency since the longest we will ever be on one Module under normal circumstances is one short week or 168 hours. The Modules are set up so that they are complementary and self-reinforcing—don't think that we have to go from **Module One** to **Module Two**, then to **Module Three**, in that order.

When we finish describing the various Modules, we'll get together on how to select the ideal sequence for our individual needs. So, although we've been going to great pains to explain in detail the nutritional qualities of each individual Module, it is only to help us understand the underlying concepts and the philosophy behind *The Diet of Diets*. As we mentioned way back in the beginning, you don't even have to think about menus or dieting or counting calories in the usual sense on this program. It's all taken care of for you. All you have to do is plug into your Module of choice, and you're bound to finish the week slimmer and happier!

Module Seven is no exception. If any Module can be said to be perfectly-balanced, **Module Seven** fits that description. It is ideally-proportioned as to nutrient content, texture, palatability, eater-satisfaction, and even color! Remember what we were saying in the first paragraph about salads? Well, **Module Seven** is a salad without the tears.

Without the tears? Oh yes. You see, the tragedy of almost every salad is contained in its name: "salad". You see, "salad", "ensalada", "insalata", "Salat" and all the rest mean "well-dosed with salt" and as we all know, salt, or sodium chloride, except in very tiny amounts can be bad news for anyone who wants to be slim, healthy, and happy. Salt can do some bad things to us and some of them happen in a very mysterious way.

For example salt can sometimes raise your blood pressure to alarming levels for no apparent reason and sometimes keep it there permanently. That's very bad news because it can easily bring on such terrible things as cerebral hemorrhages or cerebral thrombosis— sometimes known as "strokes". It can also precipitate a heart attack and a lot of other nasty things.

Like most diseases, no one knows exactly how salt acts to do you in, but we do know that excess salt has a real risk attached to it. Salt also can do something else that is always annoying and sometimes serious.

It can cause water retention. Sometimes eating salty foods can make you retain as much as two liters of water. As you know, a liter of water weighs a kilogram or just over two pounds. Two liters means that you are retaining almost five pounds of excess weight. That's bad for your body which has to deal with all that extra fluid and move it around. It also tends to accumulate in inconvenient places like your ankles, under your eyes, and around your legs and thighs.

Incidentally that problem of water retention with excess salt consumption is the way some not-so-scrupulous diet programs put something over on you. By feeding you diuretics or drugs that make you urinate a lot, they trigger a sudden dramatic weight loss that is really only a water loss.

It isn't a good idea since most diuretics work by disabling your kidneys a little so that they can't normally reabsorb water. Diuretics can be useful in some serious diseases like heart failure and water-logged lungs (pulmonary edema). But no healthy person should ever take a diuretic just to make a better impression during his morning visit to the bathroom scale. And salt can be treacherous.

For example, let's say you feel like a little snack of something salty and you munch some pretzels or potato chips.

If you don't have enough water in your body at that moment, emergency signals are sent to your brain and you suddenly feel thirsty. Then you have to drink a lot of water to attempt to dilute the salt that you have inflicted on yourself.

Once all that water pours into your tissues, it doesn't leave so easily and you become "water-logged". Each liter adds another kilogram (or 2.2 pounds) to your morning session with the unforgiving scale. Of course that extra water puts an extra load on your heart and your kidneys and that extra salt does the same. You don't need it and you shouldn't use any but the very tiniest amounts of salt in your diet.

Ideally you shouldn't add salt to your food when you cook it or when you eat it. You should banish the salt shaker from the table and use it to store papers clips on your desk top.

And you'll be amazed that you won't miss the taste of salt one bit after you have a chance to adapt to it. You see, every food that you eat has natural salt in it—sodium and chloride are two of the most common elements on earth. As you stop dumping salt into your food, you will begin to taste the natural salt in everything you eat and you will be amazed at how much better your food begins to taste.

I know what you're thinking. If this Module has something to do with salad and we want to avoid all the dangers of salt, how are we going to make a salad without salt if the whole idea of "salad" comes from the word "salt"? I'll have the answer for you in just a moment but first let's have a closer look at the basic attraction of "salad".

A lot of articles have been written, especially in the older medical journals, about the importance of eating foods in the proper combinations. Some of the concepts are based on combining an acid food with an alkaline food or eating "heat-producing" foods with "cool" foods. For the most part, this was dismissed as speculation and theory. Well, not all of it was that bad.

For example we know that amino acids have to be consumed at about the same time and in specific combinations and proportions in order to give us the benefits of eating a "complete" protein. But the problem goes much deeper. Since we actually know so very little about the effect of food on our bodies, we have to depend to a great extent on our basic instincts.

Fortunately those instincts usually guide us unerringly toward right decisions in food if we pay strict attention to what is happening. Think about it this way. Haven't you had the experience where for some reason you had a sudden craving for an apple?

I mean, you just *had* to have an apple. And when you finally got one, it tasted better than any apple you had ever eaten in your life. The same thing might have happened with a tomato, a glass of lemonade, or an egg. If we had been able to do an instant analysis of your available body stores of vitamins, minerals, protein, and carbohydrate, we would probably have found that you desperately craved exactly what you needed at that moment. Of course if you think about it, it has to be that way. Your body must steer you to develop an appetite for the nutrients you need the most. Otherwise you might run the risk of trying to live on nothing but bread and pickles or anchovy pizza and boiled zucchini.

As a matter of fact there's an interesting experiment along that line that's been done many times and in many different ways. Basically this is what it consists of.

At an orphanage or a boarding school or some similar place, the food for each meal was set out on a big table so that everyone could select exactly what they felt like eating. The choices included almost every type of food imaginable. The residents could eat anything they wanted—all desserts, all meat, all pies—it didn't matter. The groups that have been tested ranged in age from tots of three and four years old to retired folks in their seventies and eighties.

As they made their selections, nutritionists watched via closed circuit television. What they found was fascinating and very important for us to know. At first many of the selections were strange. As you might predict, most of the kiddies gorged on desserts and sweets. A lot of the grown-ups did about the same. Sometimes a person would eat nothing but meat every day at every meal. On other occasions they only wanted bread and potatoes and spaghetti. Some people ate nothing but fruit for several days. But—and this is the fascinating part—at the end of a two week period, when they analyzed the total amount of food chosen by each person almost everyone had instinctively selected the equivalent of a perfectly balanced diet!

In the final analysis, they had all been unerringly guided by their inner appetites. It's important to keep that in mind as we continue because your un-perverted taste for food is an almost completely dependable guide to exactly what your body needs.

I specified "un-perverted taste" for a very good reason. The business of food processors is to improve their financial health not your physical health. They must do everything in their power to induce you to consume their products whether they are what your body needs or not. That's why they add flavors and colors and textures that tend to fool your senses of taste, smell, and touch. For example, take a basic food like orange juice. Real orange juice contains a tremendous amount of very valuable nutrients in concentrated and readily absorbable form. But real orange juice is very expensive and perishable.

So some food processors come up with various factory-made products which look and taste like real orange juice but are cheaper to make and last much longer on the supermarket shelf. It may look like orange juice—due to its artificial coloring. It may taste like orange juice—due to its artificial flavors. It may even have some of the nutrients of orange juice—due to its synthetic vitamins. But it is not orange juice!

Now here's where the real problem comes in. This factory-fresh orange drink can fool your eyes. It can fool your nose. It can fool your taste buds. But it can't fool your enzymes! You will feel as if your craving for orange juice is satisfied but you will not get the nutrition that your body was expecting from real orange juice. After you finish your glass of the artificially-colored and artificially-flavored orange liquid you've lost your taste for oranges but you're still lacking the nutrients that impelled you to search out orange juice in the first place.

Now if this were just one example, there wouldn't be much of a problem. But the imitation orange juice story is repeated each day with dozens of vital basic foods in our modern diet. That's the real hazard of most pre-prepared and processed foods. They have "built-in taste appeal" but that only means they are carefully designed to slip by our sensory receptors and make us think that we have had the real thing.

Too often they don't have the real vitamins, pre-vitamins, co-vitamins, minerals, trace elements, enzymes, co-enzymes, and all the rest of the nutrients that we need to be vigorous and healthy. That's why it's so important on *The Diet of Diets* to concentrate on fresh wholesome unprocessed food whenever possible so that all the food you eat will do everything for you that your body is expecting. Later on if you occasionally want to play around with a little bit of recreational food like ice cream, carbonated soft drinks, and potato chips, that's up to you. But even then you should do it only in small amounts and very occasionally unless you want to get fat and start *The Diet of Diets* all over again right from the beginning.

Now let's press on to our new ideas on salads. A really tasty salad seems like it has some rare undiscovered combination of vital food elements that work together in a very specific way to please the palate and satisfy the tummy of almost everyone. Maybe it's the freshness or the combination of many different types of nutritional elements that makes the difference. But whatever it is, salads are different. And ours is going to be even more different. Because it is going to be a salad without salt.

But if the basic principle of "salad" is salt, how are we going to do it? Well, the entire idea behind *The Diet of Diets* is pioneering new concepts, breaking down old barriers, and finding new and exciting ways to accomplish our goals. **Module Seven** is not an exception to this principle.

We are going to make salads without salt that taste better than salads with salt! That means we are going to have a powerful new weapon against overweight—a salad that gives us everything we need, tastes superb, and is never never boring. In the process we are going to accomplish something unheard of in the world of dieting. We are going to—once and for all—do away with that great enemy of weight loss: *Salad fatigue!* Now let's get right down to business and get it done.

What **Module Seven** consists of is a careful selection of perfectly-balanced food elements to make the next 7 days interesting and exciting—and powerfully effective in taking off the pounds. Here is the Module in all its perfection:

BREAKFAST

One hard-boiled egg
Salad greens any type, any amount, any combination
One tomato
Coffee or tea without cream or sugar

MID-DAY

One hard-boiled egg
Salad greens, any type, any amount, any combination
One tomato
Coffee or tea without cream or sugar

TWO P.M.

One hard-boiled egg
Salad greens, any type, any amount, any combination
One tomato
Coffee or tea without cream or sugar

SUPPER TIME

One hard-boiled egg
Salad greens, any type, any amount, any combination
One tomato
Coffee or tea without cream or sugar

BED TIME

One hard-boiled egg
Salad greens, any type, any amount, any combination
One tomato
Coffee or tea without cream or sugar

NOTE: Select your choice of salad greens from the vast list of salad greens below:

1. Lettuce: head lettuce, leaf lettuce, oak leaf, Boston, iceberg, bronze leaf, etc.
2. Chicory
3. Escarole
4. Endive
5. Bok Choy—Chinese cabbage
6. Roquette
7. Romaine
8. Watercress
9. Chard
10. Garden cress
11. Dandelion greens
12. Cos
13. Mustard greens
14. New Zealand spinach
15. Purslane
16. Spinach
17. Arugula

Up 'til now things look okay, but not super-exciting, right? Well, here comes the good part. You can turbo-charge these salads with an unlimited amount of the following tremendously attractive salad dressings, each of which turns the basic ingredients into an entirely new and different meal.

Here's a baker's dozen of some of the dressings—all based on plain low fat yogurt—very low in calories and very good for us:

1. Yogurt with cucumber and celery seed
2. Yogurt with curry powder and minced garlic
3. Yogurt with herbs—minced parsley, minced chives, dried basil
4. Yogurt with horseradish
5. Yogurt with chopped olives
6. Yogurt with chopped raspberries
7. Yogurt with chopped baby shrimp

8. Yogurt with chopped mint

9. Yogurt with capers

10. Yogurt with fines herbes—oregano, rosemary, tarragon

11. Yogurt with chopped onion

12. Yogurt with chopped beets and minced watercress

13. Yogurt with chopped fresh pineapple

And in farther along you'll find even more delicious salad dressings for this Module with complete recipes. Of course, the variety doesn't stop with the dressings. You can use any salad green you wish.

By constantly combining new greens with new salad dressings you can easily have a different salad for every meal of Module Seven! And remember you can eat the hard-boiled egg on the side, or crumble it up and spread it over the salad. You can even slice the egg lengthwise, remove the yolk, mash it finely, mix it with the dressing and use it to stuff the egg. So you can see that each and every salad is a new adventure—and there are five full meals every day!

Now, how does **Module Seven** stack up nutritionally? Very nicely, that's how. Let's take a look:

First, the hard-boiled egg:

water: 73%

sodium: 112 mg

calories: 163

potassium: 129 mg

protein: 13 g

vitamin A: 1180 IU

fat: 11.5%

thiamine (vitamin B1): 0.09 mg

carbohydrate: 0.9%

riboflavin: 0.28 mg

calcium: 54 mg

niacin: 0.1 mg

iron: 2.3 mg

vitamin C: 0

phosphorus: 205 mg

Now the tomato:

water: 93%
sodium: 3 mg
calories: 22
potassium: 244 mg
protein: 1.1 g
vitamin A: 900 IU
fat: 0.2%
thiamine (vitamin B1): 0.09 mg
carbohydrate: 4.7%
riboflavin: 0.28 mg
calcium: 13 mg
niacin: 0.7 mg
iron: 0.5 mg
vitamin C: 23 mg
phosphorus: 27 mg

And finally the salad greens. Since there are minor variations among the various greens, we'll use lettuce as a typical green:

water: 95%
sodium: 9 mg
calories: 14
potassium: 264 mg
protein: 1.2 g
vitamin A: 970 IU
fat: 0.2%
thiamine (vitamin B1): 0.06 mg
carbohydrate: 2.5%
riboflavin: 0.06 mg
calcium: 35 mg
niacin: 0.3 mg
iron: 2 mg
vitamin C: 8 mg
phosphorus: 26 mg

Now let's add it all up and see what we have. For five good filling and satisfying meals, we have just about 1000 calories—provided you can manage to eat everything on the Module.

As always on *The Diet of Diets*, if you're not hungry, there is no reason to force yourself to eat. Just keep in mind that you may be hungrier tomorrow so take advantage of whatever decline in appetite you may be lucky enough to have today.

Module Seven gives us a whopping seventy-six-and-half grams of protein—almost all of it the best protein in the world. (Remember that egg protein is the "perfect protein" and the standard against which all other protein foods are measured.) We will be getting 265 milligrams of calcium—very good.

There is also 24 milligrams of iron in an ideal form—in the best possible way to eat it. Vitamin A comes in at an impressive 15,250 International Units—an opportunity to fill our Vitamin A stores to the brim. We are also getting about 270 milligrams of Vitamin C in its most absorbable form. So our "salad without salt" can only mean another week of smashing success on Module Seven of *The Diet of Diets*.

Now there's one other task remaining: on to final victory with our final and most sensational Module: **Module Eight**!

10

The Last Diet You'll Ever Need!

Well, we finally made it! Now we've been through the seven Modules and maybe we've even had a chance to try them and see how wonderfully and effortlessly they work to help us lose weight. Now there's only one other thing we need to put an end to our weight problems once and for all. We need one more Module—a Module that we can follow permanently—for the rest of our lives—that will keep us slim and trim and forever thin. That's the weak point—the Achilles Heel—of almost every diet plan.

Just think of all the weight reduction diets that you have heard about in the past. On most of them, once you lose the weight, you are on your own.

Oh, they may mumble something about "being careful" or they may offer you a stern little lecture about overeating. That makes wonderful reading but it's a lot like trying to tell an alcoholic he shouldn't drink. You agree, he agrees, you both agree. But you haven't given him anything that will help him with his problem.

Since we've traveled this far together, I'm going to walk the last mile with you, just as I promised. I'm going to give you a Module that will change your life—once and for all. I'm going to finish *The Diet of Diets* with a diet plan that is a new way of life. I'm going to leave you with a system of eating that has saved millions of lives and might very well save your life as well. Does that sound like a lot to deliver? Maybe. Ready? Here we go.

Let's start at the beginning. Our goal is to come up with a Module that will be nourishing, satisfying, and that will provide you with every nutrient that you might possibly need. That same module must have some built-in protection against over-eating so that you will never be fat again. In addition, it should make you healthier than you are now and provide protection against those terrible diseases that result from defective eating habits.

How do we find a diet like that? Well, I'll tell you how I found it. I went back in history until I found a race of people who almost never got fat. I looked for a group of people who were free from the usual nutritional diseases that wreak havoc on modern society. I looked for a group of people that almost never had heart attacks or diabetes or diverticulosis or varicose veins or hemorrhoids or cancer of the colon or appendicitis or phlebitis or *Obesity!*

These are the so-called inevitable "diseases of civilization". I searched and searched and searched for such people and—guess what? I never had to go that far back into history! Can you imagine my surprise when I found them living in our midst? They had been here with us all along! To make it even more fascinating, I didn't find just one group—I found more than half a dozen! I found people who just didn't get fat—besides not getting fat, they didn't get sick from the diseases that almost all of us take for granted.

Who are these people and where do they live and why don't they get fat and sick? Well, the whole story is in a book I wrote called *The Save-Your-Life Diet* (of course available as en e-book)—but I'm going to summarize the points that are important for our purposes here.

Quite some years ago, a group of physicians working in West Africa made some fascinating observations about the African natives whom they were treating. First, they observed that appendicitis, a disease that most people in the United States take for granted, was unknown among their African patients. In addition, their patients never had heart attacks. Not only did they never have heart attacks but they had never even heard of anyone who had a heart attack!

The other diseases that I mentioned were also unknown to them. Things like diabetes, cancer of the colon, even constipation—were just words to them. But what is most important to us is the fact that they never got fat! They ate well, sometimes as much as 2000 to 3000 calories a day and they rarely over-exerted. But their weight remained well within the range of normal. What is their secret? Their secret was bound up in one little word—the little word that can mean the difference between sickness and health, happiness and despair, slimness and obesity.

You know what I'm going to say, don't you? That word is: F-I-B-E-R. *The Save-Your-Life Diet* is none other than the *Original* high fiber diet. I should probably mention that in the years since my book was published there have been scores of imitators. (If there is any doubt in your mind simply check the date of publication of *The Save-Your-Life Diet* and the publication dates of the folks who read my book and then wrote theirs.) Not all of them have understood the medical aspects of the diet but I welcome their efforts to encourage as many people as possible to improve their way of eating.

Now let's get down to the basics. What actually is fiber? Well, the kind of fiber we're interested in is dietary fiber. If you look at the food you eat, you'll notice that there are a lot of seeds and skins and strings scattered through it. Fiber is really the chewy sinewy part of our diet. For example, it is the skin on beans and the strings in string beans and the peel of apples and the seeds in oranges and the whitish partitions that divide the segments of grapefruit and the strings in pineapple. It is the part of our diet that makes us chew—and the part that most so-called "modern" food processing gets rid of.

Dietary fiber is the part of our diet that we can't digest but we must eat if we are going to be healthy—and if we want to be slim and trim. There is virtually nothing else that we can include in our diet that will do us as much good.

I studied the diets of the Africans and the Japanese and the Indonesians and the country people of Latin America and the Bantus of Africa and all the other fiber-eaters I could find. The one thing I found they had in common was this:

They consumed more than 24 grams of unrefined fiber per day.

Their diet was principally made up of things like bananas, yams, beans, unrefined rice, potatoes, corn, and the like. The strange thing about it was that these primitive diets seemed to include all the things that the standard diet books tell us not to eat if we want to lose weight!

But then how did these primitive people manage to keep slim on their high fiber diet? *The secret was that they hardly ate any refined food at all.* You'd have to look very hard to find them eating white sugar, white flour, white rice or any other of the super-refined basic foods that most Americans consider an indispensable part of their diet. Their flour is whole grain, their rice is unpolished, and their sweeteners are natural like honey or unrefined sugar.

Their fat consumption is very low and they eat very little meat. Most of their animal protein comes from eggs, chicken, and fish and seafood. Without being aware of it they are taking advantage of the protective effect of a high fiber diet. In actual fact, if you really follow a high fiber diet, you can't overeat.

You have five fiber-filled body-guards defending you against your deadliest enemy: obesity. Here are the five ways that fiber shields you from overweight:

1. Fiber containing foods are harder to chew. Strictly from a mechanical standpoint, it's harder to eat fiber. Compare the effort it takes to eat an apple with what you have to do to down half a cup of apple sauce.

   That's why you can eat the equivalent of three apples in the form of puree but eating three full-sized raw apples in a row is a challenge for most any normal person. A high fiber diet satisfies you long before the mushy low fiber version. That's why I say, "If it's hard to chew, it's good for you!"

2. The high fiber diet is much bulkier than low fiber foods. A big bulky salad keeps you occupied much longer and is more filling than a big plate of french fries, for example.

3. The high fiber diet contains a lot of "thirsty fibers". As you chew high fiber foods, those fibers absorb a lot of water. As they absorb water, they swell and expand. By the time it hits your stomach and small intestine, a high fiber meal is big and very bulky—it gives you a satisfying and lasting feeling of "fullness" that you can never achieve on a low fiber diet.

4. It seems very likely that a diet high in fiber actually reduces the absorption of calories in the small intestine by about 10% to 15%. That means that you can probably eat a given amount of

food and get the same result as if you were eating 10% to 15% less!

5. People who regularly eat a high fiber diet excrete more fat in each bowel movement than their friends on the usual low fiber diet. How nice it is to know that there is a wonderful appetizing diet that actually helps your body to get rid of fat!

With five good high-fiber friends like that on your side, you have a head-start on overweight even before you begin!

Now let's get down to the very pleasant details of the high-fiber diet. If ever there was a weight-loss/weight-maintenance diet that was appetizing and fun to eat, this is it.

Here we go on **Module Eight**! The first item on the list is where the fun begins:

1. FRESH FRUITS AND VEGETABLES

Eat them in any amount any time. But be sure to eat them with the maximum amount of fiber intact. For example, don't peel your apples or peaches or plums. Eat the core of the pineapple and the cabbage.

Of course you're not going to eat the skin of the pineapple or the avocado—but you should eat the skin of every fruit and vegetable you possibly can.

Scrub beets and cucumbers—don't peel them. Look for ways to preserve fiber rather than discarding it. Eat your potatoes roasted with the skin on. Do everything possible to preserve as much as you can of the original fiber that Nature put into every fresh fruit and vegetable. Remember: "If it's hard to chew, it's good for you!

Don't eat canned, frozen, or otherwise processed fruits or vegetables if you can possibly avoid it. The fiber content of those products is often impaired and they may contain undesirable chemical additives.

Don't eat the rind of the watermelon (unless you pickle it!) but you should eat the seeds. You can roast them or just crunch them whole as you are enjoying the watermelon. (The Chinese have been doing that for centuries.)

If you have a nice young vegetable zucchini or squash, eat it skin and all. Personally I think you should eat the seeds of the oranges and grapefruit as well. (I always do!) These seeds contain a lot of fiber and a lot of very concentrated nutrients.

Remember that Nature entrusts the essence of the entire plant to the seed and packs it with nutrients that you will find no where else. Take a look at pumpkin seeds as compared to ordinary pumpkin [All values per 100 grams]:

	Pumpkin seed	Plain old Pumpkin
Protein:	29g	1g
Fiber:	4.9g	0.8g
Calcium:	51mg	1mg
Iron:	11.2mg	0.8mg
Phosphorus:	1144mg	44mg
Thiamine:	0.24mg	0.05mg
Riboflavin:	0.19mg	0.11mg
Niacin:	2.4mg	0.6mg

Let's just let our eyes roam over those values. The seed has twenty-nine times as much protein as the vegetable. It has 6 times as much fiber. The seeds give you two-and-a-half times as much calcium as well as 14 times the iron! You can also get 26 times as much phosphorus and 5 times as much thiamine from the seed.

If you want riboflavin (and you should!) you will get about twice as much from the seed as well as 4 times the niacin. It would almost make more sense to throw away the pumpkin and just eat the seeds! Fortunately you can have both at the same price so you should enjoy them. But don't fall into the error of throwing away the best part. And speaking of throwing away the best part, that takes us to the next item on **Module Eight**:

2. WHOLE GRAIN FLOUR

Back in about 1880 the high-fiber concept was dealt a terrible blow. That's when those wonderful old millstones were replaced by the steel roller mills. That was the signal for a big and catastrophic change in human nutrition. The precision-made steel mills made it possible to remove most of the fiber from the flour and gave a product that was snowy-white and very low in fiber. The two most valuable components of the wheat berry, the wheat germ and the wheat bran, were almost completely removed. That was a terrible tragedy. Look at the results:

Comparison of flour (including bran and wheat germ) [All values per 100 grams.]

	100% Whole Wheat	**White Flour**
Calories:	318	337
Protein:	13.2g	11.3g
Carbohydrate:	65.8mg	74.8mg
Fiber:	9.6g	3g
Iron:	4.0mg	2.2mg
Phosphorus:	340mg	130mg
Thiamine:	0.46mg	0.31mg
Riboflavin:	0.08mg	0.03mg
Niacin:	5.6mg	2mg

It just takes a glance to see what happens when they grind high fiber wheat into low fiber flour. The white flour has more calories, less protein, much less fiber, half the iron, one-third the phosphorus, half the niacin and riboflavin, and much less thiamine.

The good parts—that is the wheat germ and the bran have been removed. What happens to them? Oh, they're usually fed to pigs to make them strong. A pig won't grow well on white flour—that's only for our children and for us.

So use only whole wheat flour, stone-ground if possible. Use it for your bread and bread products you eat but also spaghetti and macaroni and every other flour-based food in your diet. I know, it's hard. You have to make an extra effort to find those special products like high fiber pasta and bread and biscuits and crackers and all the rest. A hundred years ago it was easy—it was hard to find the other kind—the white pasty starchy products. Well, believe me, it's worth the effort—not only from the standpoint of nutrition but for the way it will help you control your weight. Do your best and if you can't do it that way all the time, the next item in **Module Eight** will come to your rescue:

3. WHEAT BRAN

This is the ideal fiber supplement. Fortunately the fiber that is destined for the pigs is not lost forever. You can get it in a form quite suitable for human consumption. It is a nice wheat-colored wheat-flavored granular product with a host of wonderful qualities. First and foremost, it is a superb source of dietary fiber. Each 100 milligrams of bran contains about 44 milligrams of dietary fiber—a whopping 44% dietary fiber by weight. It is one of the most concentrated forms of fiber available and should have its place in every healthful diet. Its caloric significance is negligible since it is barely metabolized by the body. It's primary function is to give you a good healthy dose of fiber with all the benefits that brings.

You should eat at least 3 tablespoonfuls each day—more if you prefer. As a fringe benefit, it will eliminate almost any problem of constipation you have ever had—provided you remember to drink at least 10 glasses of water per day. In addition it will help if you can eat your bran mixed with plain yogurt (that's the way I take mine). Of course there are a lot of other very tasty ways to eat bran. For example, you can add it to any fruit juice or mix it with any soup or combine it with ground meat or add it to home-baked bread or many other appetizing ways that you will surely think of.

Lately other forms of bran have become "fashionable". They include oat bran and rice bran. There is nothing wrong with them, of course. They are both excellent sources of dietary fiber. On the other hand, they don't have any magical properties. They won't grow hair on a bald man or improve your golf score. If you like the way they taste, eat them by all means. But the truth is that all grain brans are *just about the same* in the value of fiber they add to your diet.

The groups of people who naturally eat high-fiber diets generally consume about 24 grams of fiber a day. The average low-fiber city-dweller eats about six grams a day—that leaves a fiber deficit of about eighteen grams of fiber every twenty-four hours. You can make up a lot of that deficit simply by switching to a high-fiber diet but to be absolutely sure that you're getting enough fiber it make sense to add at least three tablespoons of bran to your daily diet. (Since your digestive system is used to a low fiber diet, at first you may find the high fiber diet and the bran a little gassy. Just reduce the amount of bran and raise it slowly.)

4. WHOLE GRAIN CEREALS

There's a whole world out there of wonderful appetizing and nutritious cereals just waiting to be eaten. They include such things as unpolished barley, cracked wheat (sometimes called "bulgur"), unpolished rice, whole grain buckwheat, whole grain oats, and whole grain corn meal. They belong in everyone's diet—and they were there for about 500,000 years until modern food processing took them away from us a short 100 years ago. It's about time to bring them back. By the way, if you observe carefully you will notice that most fat people don't eat these grains—they don't even know that they exist! If they did, they probably wouldn't be nearly as fat.

5. HIGH FIBER SNACK FOODS

This is one of the best and most appetizing additions you can make to your diet. Instead of sweets and ice cream and low fiber cakes and biscuits, you can enjoy far more healthful snacks such as nuts, popcorn, sunflower seeds, our old friend the pumpkin seeds, dried fruit, raisins, and even toasted soybeans. You'll find them all to be very filling, high in fiber and unlikely to add so much as an ounce to your weight.

There's one other little detail that you should know about. Believe it or not, there are some people in this world who don't like the high fiber diet. As a matter of fact, they hate it! It doesn't take a genius to figure out who those folks might be. They're usually the ones who want you to eat white sugar and white flour and white rice—and all the rest. As a result some rather strange articles have appeared warning of dire consequences if you dare to eat high fiber foods. One of the bad things that is supposed to happen is that fiber will somehow "scratch" your stomach! That's about as cuckoo as can be! As soon as fiber—including bran—comes in contact with water, it forms a kind of gel-like mass that couldn't scratch anything!

Another fairy tale that is supposed to scare you away from fiber is the goblin of "phytic acid"! According to the gobbledy-gook that surrounds that one, a sinister substance known as "phytic acid", found in whole wheat bread, eats up all your calcium and will ultimately leave you with the bone structure of an octopus! That's one of the silliest things that has every been written in the field of nutrition!

Unrefined wheat flour does have some phytic acid in it— fortunately for us. And phytic acid does tie up a small amount of the calcium in your blood. That's why people who eat high fiber diets have virtually no trouble with calcium kidney stones! The loose calcium in your bloodstream that can only make trouble is soaked up by the phytic acid. But since phytic acid is destroyed by the yeast in the bread, your chances of having any problem as a result are about the same as being run over by a kangaroo in downtown Philadelphia while riding a giraffe and carrying a porcupine under each arm. Okay? Now let's talk about serious things.

There are some foods you want to be sure not to eat on **Module Eight**. Here they are in summarized form. Actually the list is not hard to remember since it is the mirror image of the high fiber foods that we've just gone over:

1. **White Foods**—that includes white flour, white rice and white sugar. These products are all de-nutrified and have no place in **Module Eight**.

   Don't be fooled by the fact that some of them may be advertised as "enriched". Generally that amounts to removing about 24 important nutrients and partially replacing two or three. Just ask yourself this question, "If they didn't do anything bad to the food why did they have to enrich it?". I had a friend who used to say: "The whiter the bread, the sooner you're dead!"

2. **Processed Foods**—That includes everything that is imitation, artificial, synthetic and otherwise factory-fresh. Almost all processed foods are processed either to make them able to stand long months of storage before they are sold or to make them seem like better quality natural foods. In the process they usually become quite expensive since someone has to pay for all that processing—not to mention those layers of fancy packaging, shiny labels, and advertising. As you probably have noticed, no one takes prime time television ads for fresh lettuce or wonderful crisp cabbages …

3. **Canned, Frozen, Pre-mixed and otherwise Pre-packaged Products**—None of these manipulations increases the true nutritional value of food although it does increase the cost. If you are going to concentrate on fresh fruits and vegetables, you want to make your money go as far as possible so don't spend it on high technology processes that don't really add anything to what your body is going to get from the food.

There are also a couple of "take-it-easy" areas on the high-fiber diet. These are foods that you don't have to give up but you don't want them to overwhelm your diet either:

4. **Meat**—I'm not going to make you into a vegetarian against your will—nothing of the sort. But if you eat a lot of meat you will find that it displaces the fiber from your diet. Remember that the only kind of fiber that benefits you is vegetable fiber. The animal fibers in meat offer no dietary advantages whatsoever. Try and cut down on your meat consumption gradually and replace it with the best quality fruits and vegetables and grains that you can find. Instead of eating your meat in massive quantities by itself, try combining it with other foods in pasta dishes, casseroles, salads, and the like.
You'll be amazed at how good meat tastes when you have other ingredients to bring out its true flavor. You will also find that you will save a lot of money on food at the same time you are eating better! After all, meat is one of the most expensive items on your shopping list. (And my vegetarian friends point out, it is also the cadaver of a dead animal.)

5. **Dairy Products**—They are not the same hazard that meat is since they are not nearly as filling. You just want to make sure that they don't displace vegetable fiber from your diet.
The same is true of eggs although here the risk is small since eggs don't occupy a big place in the diet of the average adult. You can smooth everything out nicely if you combine cheese and eggs with high-fiber foods such as whole-grain bread and breading and similar items. And you'll find that it makes everything taste better in the process! Remember milk and

yogurt and cheese helped us a lot along the way—we can still eat them but now in moderation.

6. **Alcohol**—Drinks are a hazard on any reducing diet but if they replace fiber on **Module Eight** they are a double hazard. But how can drinks replace fiber? Easy. Remember that alcohol is a refined carbohydrate and after a couple of bottles of beer you don't want a nice thick slice of whole wheat bread or a couple of nice crisp apples. Your appetite for carbohydrate is satiated and you are more likely to go for fiber-less protein instead. Like maybe a good thick steak? The same is true for a martini or a highball or a couple of glasses of wine. So drink if you like, but take it easy and remember that if you want to keep all the hard-earned benefits of *The Diet of Diets*, fiber comes first!

7. **Chicken, Fish and Seafood**—These are lesser hazards since you are not likely to let them displace very much of your fiber but just keep an eye on your consumption and try to combine these dishes with high fiber foods such as bread and salads and the like.

I think that's all you need to know about the basic concepts of **Module Eight**. Now let's have a look at some sample menus that will amaze and delight you:

BREAKFAST

Raw apple with skin
Any whole grain cereal (pick one made without refined sugar) with milk and sliced bananas
Whole wheat toast
Tea or coffee—use raw honey instead of sugar— add milk as desired

LUNCH

Two small slices Roast Beef
Baked potato with skin intact
Fresh green beans
Green salad

Fresh strawberries
Tea or coffee—use raw honey instead of sugar—add milk
as desired

DINNER

Homemade vegetable soup
Broiled chicken
Fresh green beans
Fresh corn
High fiber rice pudding
Tea or coffee—use raw honey instead of sugar—add milk
as desired

BED TIME SNACK

Dish of fresh raspberries

There are some very nice recipes for hundreds of genuine high-fiber dishes in a book I wrote. It's called *The Save-Your-Life Diet High Fiber Cook Book* and is full of simple and very tasty recipes. Let me run through another day's menu and we'll be ready to move on to the next chapter. Here we go:

BREAKFAST

Cheese omelet
Whole grain rye crackers
Two fresh oranges sliced—with coconut sprinkled over the
top
Tea or coffee—use raw honey instead of sugar—add milk
as desired

LUNCH

Whole wheat spaghetti with cheese and tomato sauce
Italian green salad
Bunch of red grapes
Tea or coffee—use raw honey instead of sugar—add milk
as desired

DINNER

Curried shrimp on a bed of unpolished rice
Mango chutney
Raw spinach salad
Baked eggplant
Tea or coffee—use raw honey instead of sugar—add milk
as desired

BED TIME SNACK

A bowl of piping-hot freshly-popped popcorn

Because there are so many possibilities to choose from on **Module Eight,** you can make up hundreds of menus to perfectly suit your own tastes. I think you'll find it interesting and exciting.

Module Eight is really a Module for a lifetime. It's the way that human beings should eat—as a matter of fact, they never should have stopped eating that way! With a little practice, you will find that it's easy to stick with the Module—at work on vacation when you're eating out—just about anywhere and under any circumstances. What happens if you start to put on weight? Well, if you're following **Module Eight** the way you should, that should never happen. But we know that this a far from perfect world and accidents do happen. So be sure to continue to weigh yourself every morning of your life and when you see that you have crept three pounds over your normal weight, put *The Diet of Diets Emergency Plan* into action. Immediately, select the *The Diet of Diets* Module that you liked the best and go back on it for seven days.

You should easily take off those thirty-six terrible ounces and find yourself right back where you want to be. But be sure not to neglect this vitally important detail. Remember, when you got fat before, you didn't gain a hundred pounds overnight. You puffed up a pound or two at a time. So three pounds of weight gain is ample warning and you really must take it seriously. After all, you don't ever want to be fat again, do you?

Now let's move on to the next chapter where we will tie together some important final details.

11

Some Simple And Delicious Recipes

Remember back there when I promised you some "Simple and Delicious Recipes"? Well as you've noticed I always keep my promises. This is the Chapter where we actually "Tie the ribbons on …" That's when we gather together all the various little details that go along with a successful diet to make *The Diet of Diets* the most enjoyable and rewarding diet that you have ever followed. Not only will we come through with some "simply delicious" recipes, but we'll give you a Module-by-Module summary to wrap things up.

But first, let's take a moment for a short explanation. In most of the popular fad diets, usually written by folks who have neither training nor experience in medicine nor nutrition, you'll see a lot of so-called "diet" foods. These are usually chemical combinations that no one ever heard of until one day they jumped out of the laboratory test-tubes.

That includes things like "diet" soft drinks and imitation sweeteners and sugar substitutes. You won't see any of those chemicals in *The Diet of Diets*. Here's why:

"Eat all the imitation artificial *what-ever-you-call-it* you want and you'll never get fat!"

I don't think anyone should consume a food product that hasn't been in use at least a hundred years or so. Let someone else try it for the first century and then I can recommend it to the people I care about the most—my readers.

There's another important point that none of the amateur diet-book-writers seems to understand either. If you are trying to lose weight permanently, it is scientifically sensible to re-educate your eating habits. The only permanent solution to the real menace of obesity is to learn to eat naturally like a normal human being—for the rest of your life. The only diet that offers that to everyone is *The Diet of Diets* and it's yours for the asking. Enjoy it.

Now let's get down to some of the exciting details of the individual modules. In **Module One**, you should be using a lot of mayonnaise— unless of course you don't like mayonnaise. In that case, I'll give you a substitute that will make you just as happy. I would prefer to see you making your own mayonnaise since some of the commercial mayonnaise products have funny things like starch—and worse—in them. If you'll just take a little extra effort, you will be well rewarded in better results on **Module One**. Here's the recipe:

REAL MAYONNAISE

2 tbsp. lemon juice
1 cup olive oil (if you don't care for olive oil, use some other oil but olive is best!)
1 raw egg
1 tsp. dry mustard
Put all the ingredients except the oil in a blender or food processor. Turn it on to high speed. Slowly pour the oil in a very thin stream or drop by drop. It should make a nice smooth mayonnaise. If it doesn't, don't worry—just use it on a green salad as a Caesar dressing. It will taste fine. Notice there is no salt in this recipe. That's why the lemon juice and mustard are important.

What if you can't even spare the three minutes that this takes? Then try this recipe for instant "almost mayonnaise":

ALMOST MAYONNAISE

Just mix the oil and lemon juice and toss in the raw egg. Then whip it up with a fork or a whisk. You'll have a very tasty dressing in seconds! No salt, no sugar, no flour. It may not look like what you see on TV but it will be excellent quality and much cheaper than the store-bought kind.

Speaking of salads, please don't be afraid of garlic. The smell may be a little strange to you but it will not turn your true friends against you and it will confuse your enemies. Garlic is a noble spice and will actually help you feel satisfied on your diet.

Don't ask me why—nobody knows. But garlic does add to the feeling of fullness during a meal. Here's the secret of eating garlic. Use it on your salads! Fresh green vegetables contain chlorophyll and chlorophyll completely dissipates the odor of garlic. Try it and you'll be amazed!

Try to stay away from the vegetables and fruit if you can on **Module One** because it will make a difference in the speed and amount of your weight loss. You will notice there is a wonderful dish called, "Omelet Aux Fines Herbes". You can select your own "fines herbes" and just mix them in with the omelet ingredients before you start to make your omelet.

You can use a mixture of oregano, rosemary, thyme, and chervil— all fresh or in dried form—or really any combination you like. As far as the omelets are concerned, the sky is the limit just as long as you stick to the basic idea of the diet. You can have chicken omelets, meat omelets, seafood omelets, or any other type of omelet that occurs to you as long as it in line with the basic concept of that specific Module.

On **Module Two** is where you can let your imagination and creativity run riot. Remember that you can use any fruit and any vegetable in the amounts indicated just so long as it is fresh. A sweetish fruit is nice on top of your rice for breakfast with something a little more tart for lunch and something substantial for dinner. The same holds true for the vegetable portion of this Module. Try a light vegetable for breakfast, a moderate one for lunch and something a little more bracing for dinner. Of course, these are only suggestions. You may prefer to do it exactly the opposite way—in which case that's the perfect way for you! So try it and see what fits in best with your own personal tastes.

When you get to **Module Three**, your menu-planning worries are over. Just grab your bunch of bananas and your jug of skimmed milk and you're light as a feather. As they used to say on television, "No mess, no fuss, no bother!"

Module Four takes just the tiniest bit of trickery but it's well worth it. This is where we're trying to get rid of the last drop of fat in our Module. But as you've noticed, we still want to do a little bit of frying—you know, it makes a diet taste better. There are two superb ways to fry without fat: high-technology and low technology. There is also a way to fry almost without fat.

The high technology fry-without-fat system is to use one of those fancy plastic-lined frying pans that won't let the food stick to it. Yes, Teflon is a plastic. (Isn't everything in this world getting to be plastic?) I don't have to tell you how to use non-stick pans—the instructions come right along with the little beauties.

Personally I like the low technology method much better. It involves a plain old black cast-iron frying pan—hopefully one that's been in the family for many years. It should have done a lot of frying in its day and since cast iron is porous—you knew that!—it absorbs oil over the years. So you don't really have to add any oil to cook in it. Maybe just wipe a cloth barely dampened in oil over the bottom and sides each time before you cook in it to be super-sure. What you never want to do is wash out a cast iron pan. That takes all the oil out that has soaked in over the years and will probably make your family heirloom rust away! Washing a cast iron pan is tantamount to scratching a Teflon utensil—the kitchen equivalent of a capital offense!

What do you do if you don't have a black cast iron pan that has been handed down from the time of the Second Voyage of Columbus? Don't be concerned in the least. You can make up your own. Just pop over to your local Shopping Center and buy the nicest black cast iron frying pan that you can find. As soon as you get it home from the store wash it well with soap and water. (This will be the first and last time you are going to do this, so do it thoroughly.) Then rinse and dry it carefully and cover the bottom and sides with a thin layer of the kind of oil you are going to use the most—olive oil, corn oil, safflower—whatever you prefer. Then put the pan into a warm oven—say about 200°F—and leave it there an hour or two until all the oil is absorbed. Repeat the oil treatment—but not the washing—once or twice more and you have an almost instant heirloom. You can then cook most anything in it if you keep the heat within reasonable limits and wipe it out with the tiniest amount of oil each time you use it. And of course, you won't be washing it after use. Just take out whatever you've cooked and wipe the inside clean with an oil-anointed cloth. It's a simple and healthful and elegant way of doing it.

There are also "spray-on" substances that you can use for "fat-free" frying. They are usually lecithin – derived from soy beans and they work pretty well. You can use them if you like them.

I'm sure you noticed that I included "Broiled Chicken With Herb Sauce" in one of the menu plans. It's a great dish with many variations that you yourself will think of simply by varying the amount and quantity of spices. Here's the basic recipe:

BROILED CHICKEN WITH HERB SAUCE

Take one whole broiling chicken and broil it the way you usually do. While it's cooking whip up the following sauce:

½ Cup lemon juice

¼ Cup finely chopped parsley

½ tsp. dried Basil

2 tomatoes finely chopped

¼ tsp. black pepper (preferably freshly ground)

¼ tsp. fennel seed

1 small onion, finely minced

Put all the ingredients in a blender or food processor and blend briefly at low speed—just enough to break up the solid ingredients. Then simmer slowly for 15 minutes on low heat. When the chicken is cooked, quickly cut it into individual pieces and pour the hot sauce over it. Make plenty because it will vanish in an instant!

Now on to the "Eggplant and Tomato Casserole with Oriental Spices". Here's the simple and succulent recipe for that one:

EGGPLANT AND TOMATO CASSEROLE WITH ORIENTAL SPICES

1 eggplant cut into approximately one inch cubes

2 tomatoes cut about the same size

1 small onion chopped

2 tsp. ground coriander

1 tsp. ground turmeric

½ tsp. cumin powder

¼ cup apple cider vinegar

¼ cup water

Mix all the ingredients well, simmer slowly one-half hour on medium-low heat. Serve immediately. I'm sure you'll be back for second helpings of that wonderful eggplant-tomato-onion dish!

Now here's another very nice **Module Three** recipe:

COLESLAW WITH CIDER VINEGAR AND FRESH GRAPES

Slice very fine or chop one very fresh green cabbage (Here's a trick I use that you might like. Cut the cabbage into quarters and fill your blender jar half way with cold water. Drop the cabbage quarters in and blend—with the top on! When the cabbage is nicely sliced up, pour the entire contents into a strainer and drain the water away. Easy, fast, and you'll never slice a finger this way!)

Then take ½ cup of good cider vinegar, ½ cup of water, and 1 tablespoon of honey. Blend it together and mix it with the sliced-up cabbage. Add two good tablespoons of celery seed—more or less if you like—and toss it all together. Garnish it with a big handful of fresh green tart grapes for each person. The combination of flavors here is really something you have to taste for yourself!

I owe you one more recipe on this Module and with great pleasure, here it is:

BEETS AND WATERCRESS MARINADE

4 medium cooked beets, sliced

¼ cup vinegar

¼ cup water

½ cup finely chopped watercress

2 tbsp. very finely minced onion

1 tbsp. honey

Mix all the ingredients except the beets. Blend thoroughly—preferably in a blender or food processor. Pour over the sliced beets and refrigerate at least 3 hours. I made this recipe for 4 beets but honestly, once you taste this combination, I think you will want at least twice as much.

There's not much in the way of recipes in **Module Six**. It's just a matter of getting the best quality buttermilk and the best quality cottage cheese you can find. Even if you have to go a bit out of your way to do it, it's more than worthwhile because you deserve the best.

Now we come to **Module Seven** and that's where I owe you a lot of recipes for a lot of wonderfully appetizing salad dressings. But don't worry—it's only one basic recipe and once you master it—in about 3 minutes—you can make endless combinations on your own. Pretty soon you'll be sending me recipes!

The basic idea in this Module is to provide an attractive choice of salad dressings to make the various salads as interesting as possible. The problem, of course, is that most commercial salad dressings are a combination of an acid—lemon juice or vinegar—and an oil—olive oil, corn oil, etc. And of course, there's that massive dose of salt that we have mentioned so often. The solution that we are going to use is ideal—kick out the salt but not the taste of salt, add a microscopic amount of fat, and a whopping dose of garden-fresh flavor. What's the secret? Yogurt is the secret.

As you know, yogurt is milk that has been seeded with a culture of a very special kind of bacteria called "lactobacillus acidophilus". The translation from Latin to English tells it all: "a bacteria that grows in milk and likes a slightly acidic environment". The lacto-bacillus acidophilus bacteria is a very interesting one. It is the main bacteria in the large intestine of most normal people and there is strong evidence that it provides protection against cancer. It's also been discovered that diets that are low in fiber and high in meat content reduce the amount of lactobacillus acidophilus bacteria that a person has. There's much more to the exciting story of yogurt than that, but for the moment, that's enough.

Most commercial yogurt is made from partly skimmed milk and has a fat content that runs about 1½% or less. The lemon juice that we are going to use—fresh lemon juice please—tricks our taste buds into thinking that we are tasting something salty. The explanation is fascinating. We have very special sensors for each type of taste-stimulation gathered in special areas of our mouths. It turns out that the receptors for the acidy flavors are very close to the receptors for the salty flavors and the acid flavor of freshly-squeezed lemon juice is just enough to overwhelm the salty receptors and make us think we are eating salt! It's a nice little trick that we can use to our advantage. Here's the basic recipe:

YOGURT SALAD DRESSING

1 cup plain low-fat yogurt (unsweetened and unflavored)
⅛ cup freshly-squeezed lemon juice (1 ounce)
Mix well until the two ingredients are completely blended.
Then add one or more of any of the following:

1. ½ cup finely chopped cucumber and 1 tsp. celery seed.
2. 1 tablespoon curry powder—make sure that the curry powder you use does not have any salt in it!
3. ¼ to ½ cup of freshly chopped herbs—parsley, minced chives, basil.
4. 1 to 3 tablespoons of horseradish—be sure it doesn't have salt.
5. ¼ cup chopped olives—unsalted. Try and use the fresh black olives.
6. ¼ cup fresh raspberries—cut up.
7. ½ cup chopped baby shrimp—please try and use fresh shrimp.
8. ½ cup finely chopped fresh mint.
9. ¼ cup capers—make sure to wash all the salt from them.
10. ½ teaspoon fines herbes—oregano, rosemary, tarragon. If you're lucky enough to be able to get these fresh, use one teaspoon each and you'll be so delighted that you'll use this dressing over and over again.
11. ⅛ to ¼ cup chopped onion—for onion lovers.

12. ⅛ to ¼ cup very finely chopped beets and minced watercress—you can add a dash of horseradish to this appetizing mixture if you like.

13. ¼ cup chopped fresh pineapple.

14. 2 hard-boiled egg yolks mashed together with the yogurt and lemon juice combination.

15. ½ to 1 tablespoon of powdered garlic—for garlic lovers. Be sure that you use pure powdered garlic and not "garlic salt"—that's a mixture of some garlic and a lot of salt.

16. ½ cup fresh chopped strawberries.

Well, we've come to the end of our journey together. But that doesn't mean that we have to lose touch with each other forever. Please write to me, at author@davidreubenmd.com if there's anything that you want me to know about. And I have a feeling that we'll meet each other again before too long. Until then, my very warmest wishes for your continued and ever-increasing health and happiness.